ALLERGIES *and* CANDIDA WITH THE PHYSICIST'S RAPID *SOLUTION*

FOURTH EDITION

INCLUDING THE ANSWER TO...

THE CHRONIC FATIGUE SYNDROME

FIBROMYALGIA

MULTIPLE CHEMICAL SENSITIVITIES

ENVIRONMENTAL ILLNESS

CHRONIC ILLNESS

LEARNING DISORDERS

PARASITOSIS

D0780917

ACKNOWLEDGEMENTS

I thank Professor Max Dresden for having taught me Science. When the time came, this was all I had to separate the truth from the medical morass. Fortunately, it was enough; it will always be enough. Thanks to Albert Rowe, M.D. and Albert Rowe, Jr., M.D., whose Allergy text helped me to save my life. And likewise to those allergists and ecologists who found the first half of the puzzle. And to my father who helped me when no one else would.

For research support, I thank Fred Shull, M.D. Thanks also to Emmanuel Viscussi, M.D., Harvey Maltz, D.D.S., and Ellen Whooley. Special thanks to the following people. Dr. John Wright for the lovely foreword and Ken Vatter for the fine art work.

My thanks to the early kinesiologists who helped lay the framework for me to solve the second half of the puzzle.

My deepest thanks to the following people. Joan Hulse, for encouraging me to form the H.E.B.S. program and for selflessly sponsoring it. Renée Waller, for insisting on paying an (unbeknownst-to-her disabled) physicist for a telephone "consultation" on ecology and nutrition and for sponsoring the first in-house lecture back in 1980. This launched my new career. All who've been helped by these methods owes more to Renée than they may ever know.

And finally to Australian cover model, Rose Rochford— the loveliest and most beautiful girl in the world for having gone through several hours with an amateur, New York photographer while she had pneumonia; and for offering me the entire contents of her piggy bank when she (mistakenly) thought I had run out of money. Some physicists speculate that consciousness (and language) can act as an observer and so alter the Universe. If there is any truth in this, then her Mom must have somehow known—in contradistinction to Shakespeare—that this one would be so lovely and beautiful that she could *only* be called... Rose.

ALLERGIES*and* CANDIDA WITH THE PHYSICIST'S RAPID *SOLUTION*
FOURTH EDITION

TOWARDS A SCIENCE OF HEALING
VOL. I

By Prof. STEVEN ROCHLITZ

FOREWORD BY JOHN WRIGHT, M.D.

ARTWORK BY KEN VATTER

HUMAN ECOLOGY BALANCING SCIENCE
PUBLISHING THAT UNITES SCIENCE & HEALING

Sedona, Arizona

ALLERGIES *and* CANDIDA
WITH THE PHYSICIST'S RAPID
SOLUTION, Fourth Edition
TOWARDS A SCIENCE OF HEALING, VOL. I
By Prof. Steven Rochlitz

© Copyright 2000 by Steven Rochlitz
Published by Human Ecology Balancing Science
P.O. Box 21091   Sedona, AZ 86341 USA
ISBN: 0-945262-48-5
Library of Congress Catalog Card Number: 91-3199
Printed in the USA Earlier editions copyright: 1988, 1989, 1991, 1993, 1995, 1997, 1999

Warning-Disclaimer
This book is designed to provide accurate, research information in regard to the
subject matter covered. It is not intended to offer medical, psychological or other
professional services. For medical and psychological diagnosing, prescribing
and treatment, consult a licensed professional. The author and publisher shall
have neither liability nor responsibility to any person or entity with respect to
any alleged loss or damage alleged to be caused directly or indirectly by the
information contained in this book.

Library of Congress Cataloging-in-Publication Data

Rochlitz, Steven.
    Allergies and candida : with the physicist's rapid solution / by
Steven Rochlitz : foreword by John Wright : artwork by Ken Vatter. -
    p.   cm.
    Includes bibliographical references and index.
    Contents: v. 1. Towards a science of healing.
    ISBN 0-945262-20-5 (v. 1). —ISBN 0-945262-21-3 (pbk. : v. 1)
    1. Allergy—Alternative treatment.   2. Candidiasis—Alternative
treatment.   3. Applied kinesiology.   I. Title.
RC585.R63   1991
616.97'06—dc20   91-3199

TABLE OF CONTENTS

FOREWORD

I suppose that everyone has a turning point in their career when some startling change takes place which inspires and stimulates a new wave of thought and a different exciting change of direction. This important moment occurred for me in November 1985 when I attended a seminar given by Steven Rochlitz in Melbourne, Australia.

At that time of my 12 year medical career in General Practice, I was puzzled and frustrated by some of the inadequacies of my conventional medical teaching in dealing with a significant number of patients. Those who supposedly had nothing wrong with them for all blood tests, X-rays, C.A.T. scans, etc., were normal yet they were not well and the patient knew it. And then there were those who had been told they will never be cured and that they must take drug therapy for the rest of their lives.

How exciting then to be taught a new technique that could demonstrate that their bodies were totally out of balance and therefore they were sick. The delight on the faces of patients is heartwarming, for it vindicates their belief that something is wrong with their bodies and that someone realizes their predicament and can show their illness to them. Even more rewarding is the ability to offer help in a positive way, for by following the technique of Steven Rochlitz in balancing the body, the patient's system is readjusted so that it can start to function normally again and so give it the ability to help cure itself.

No two balances are the same, as no two bodies are similar, and no two bodies become out of balance in the same way so each balance is a challenge and becomes a very personalized form of therapy, specific to each patient. After a balance is achieved, and if a good diet is maintained and medication is kept to the absolute minimum (or in most cases stopped), the results are quite stunning.

In my practice, over the past six months, I have been able to achieve some notable successes and even cures.

Some patients after a total balance have ceased all anti-hypertensive therapy and remained normotensive, have ceased antidepressants, hypnotics, sedatives and remained happy, have ceased diuretics and remained well, have recovered from asthma, hay fever, food allergies, irritable bowel symptoms, arthritis, vertigo, learning disorders, fatigue and eczema. They have regrown hair, regained concentration, have regained normal menstrual cycles, have lost weight, have performed better at sports and most regained energy, happiness and vitality. This balance will not cure all illness and is not the total panacea for problems but without the balance the body will not have a chance to heal itself.

With this book, the reader will now be able to overcome all the complaints I have outlined above. As for my medical colleagues, I hope in time the profession will accept Rochlitz' balancing methods and that they can be taught to all keen and enthusiastic medical students. In this way, many costs of drug therapy can be saved, many patients will feel better and remain well, and the doctor will be able to treat the illness and prevent its reoccurrence rather than treat, retreat, retreat, retreat and retreat. Thank you Steve for your inspired work.

John Wright, M.D.

To

Dan Everts,
Friend

PREFACE TO THE FOURTH EDITION

Allergies, Candida, Parasites, Chronic Fatigue Syndrome, Fibromyalgia, Multiple Chemical Sensitivities, Environmental Illness, or chronic illness in general—*the answers have always been in this book*—which has now lasted for thirteen years, four editions, and two millenia!

It was necessary to have a fourth edition for the following reasons. Shortly after the third ediition came out in 1991, it became clear to this author that Candidiasis was—80-90 per cent of the time—either due to an initial parasitosis; or was in fact non-existent. That is, the person suffers from parasitosis and not Candidiasis.

We revised the third edition several times to reflect this knowledge, but it was high time to change many pages in the text. Because we had to make so many changes and additions to the text and were limited by book manufacturing principles, this edition's pages may not have uniform text. We believe the sacrifice in appearance is worth the new knowledge contained in this fourth edition. Much of the book was rewritten.

There are many new or revised topics included besides all the new references to Protozoan parasites throughout. These include discussions of Helicobacter pylori bacterium, Morton's neuroma as cause of gait reflex problems, "zappers" combatting chronic viruses, the cause of "psychological reversal," weather sensitivity revised, and more.

I give my continued thanks to Cathy Thompson for repeatedly referring her own clients to me; to Alexander Reichl for his integrity and intelligence so rare in the world of kinesiology; and to Helga Kaufmann. I now thank Sophia Wu and Hanspeter Brunner. I would like to thank Helen Schiller for the lovely, new epilogue. The wisdom she displayed in travelling from the east coast to Arizona with two young babies by herself is remarkable. That she stayed for nine days until her babies were well is further proof of her trust and determination.

A very, special thanks to Dan Everts—to whom this book is dedicated—for his friendship and for helping me to relocate and for his generosity.

Prof. Steven Rochlitz
Sedona, AZ
January, 2000

PREFACE TO THE THIRD EDITION

In this edition, we have done several things. First we have, of course, updated the book with new findings. We have also included: a summary, new listings that also succinctly summarize some of our findings, a description of what the reader needs to do *now*, and what the reader needs to eat (and not eat) *now*. These are found in the new Appendix—F.

Next we have changed and improved many of the photos in this book. There are other minor changes throughout. This edition of *Allergies and Candida: With The Physicist's Rapid Solution* is now available in a limited, autographed hard cover version! These last two editions have been printed on the highest quality, recycled paper with soy ink used again.

We want to thank Gloria Vivo, Dan Everts, Joe Connolly, Cathy Thompson, Robert Sampson, M.D., and Tim Kaufmann, Helga Kaufmann and Alexander Reichl of Germany for their support. We thank all those who have made this book and its methods a huge success with 50,000 copies now in print!

Though the third edition first appeared in 1991, the text has been revised in 1993, 1995, 1997 and here in the 1999 version. The last two revised third editions emphasize that parasitosis is often the cause of chronic fatigue/chronic illness/food and chemical allergies and Candidiasis is often secondary to amoebiasis or giardiasis or other parasitosis. Finally, the reader is advised to read the next two prefaces for hints on how to read this book.

Prof. Steve Rochlitz
Sedona, AZ
January, 1999

PREFACE TO THE SECOND EDITION

Welcome to the revised, expanded, improved second edition of, what many of our readers have said, is the best health book of the decade. We thank all the first edition readers who wrote to us with their congratulations. Our readers will find hundreds of additions to the text in this edition. We have also made numerous typographic changes and improvements here in the second edition of **ALLERGIES AND CANDIDA.** The text is larger and even more readable. Kinesiological "recipes" and all compilations (of symptoms, causes, etc.) are listed in a clearer, vertical format and the reader is urged (in bold) to perform them immediately upon first reading!

We've added a new Appendix (E) which you can refer to at anytime if you forget what any abbreviation stands for. Footnote references that have been added in this edition are noted by a superscript letter instead of a number so readers of the first edition can trace the new references. We have also added several chapters and have broken up the large allergy chapter. There are now separate chapters on weight loss science, addictions—including alcoholism, the immune system, hypoglycemia, energy and vitamin allergy and an epilogue which depicts how a reader of the first edition was able to get herself well. Thanks to Harvey Maltz, DDS for suggesting the subtitle that we have adopted. The reader should be advised that the subtitle—*"THE PHYSICIST'S RAPID SOLUTION"*— has two components. A virtually immediate one (kinesiological, energy balancing of the body's electrical systems) and the longer (ecological) component.

We want to say thanks to all the healers, educators and physicians who have purchased so many first edition books, directly from us, to offer to their patients and clients.

The new reader is advised to read the following preface to the first edition. It contains many helpful tips on how to read this book. You should first peruse the book and the table of contents. Decide for yourself what you want to read first. (Many people are spurred on by first reading the "Science, Medicine & Society" and the "Psychology" chapters.) The book is written in the following order. First detailed are the causes of most health complaints today. Then, what follows is really the first, self-help manual. So, if you can't wait to be well—to immediately improve your physical and mental well-being—you can skip to the kinesiology section first.

Steven Rochlitz
New York,
August, 1989

PREFACE TO THE FIRST EDITION

Welcome to the future! Yes, it was necessary to create *"THE PHYSICIST'S RAPID SOLUTION"* to the devastating "20th Century Disease" of Universal Allergies and Candidiasis. What you are about to read is the first "how-to" wellness manual for the ecologically ill and those that wish to never become ecologically ill. (Ecological illness refers to allergies, Candidiasis [a Candida or yeast problem] and related ills. We will refer to this term throughout the book.) Not only is this the first book to cover both Allergies *and* Candida; it also contains step-by-step instructions on how to test and balance many of the underlying imbalances that have kept (until now) so many in an unwell state. Henceforth, books on Allergies or Candida, if they are not to be obsolete, should include similar methodologies. This book makes the basic tools and simple theory of the *PHYSICIST'S RAPID SOLUTION* available to everyone.

This book is written for all Allergy and Candida sufferers and the practitioners who treat them. And yes, you can balance yourself and remain well. In fact, all the exercise and touch corrections in this book, are designed to allow the reader to correct himself, if need be.

Chapter 1 details how a physicist was forced to learn and create the methods of this book to save his life and to get well. Chapters 2-8 reveal the intricacies of allergies, Candidiasis and related ecological matters. We have made these chapters succinct, up-to-date, complete, yet lucid. The next four chapters cover the new Science of Kinesiology or Muscle Biofeedback Testing (**MBT**) and Energy Balancing—the missing link in the physicist's rapid solution. This is the other side of the coin in our two-model approach to health. Throughout, we stress that it is not a substitute for medical testing and treatment, rather it is complementary, yet crucial, if wellness is to be attained. This approach is based on ancient (and proven) Chinese acupuncture theory with significant modern innovations. Muscle testing and balancing are clearly the unstoppable wave of the future. We hope after reading this book, every ecologically-oriented physician will seek to add the services of an expert kinesiologist to his staff. This second section demonstrates how easily MBT can uncover both sensitivities and energy impediments that must be unblocked before wellness can be attained.

After showing the reader how to use MBT, we reveal that dyslexia is an ecological illness (**E.I.**) and is found in virtually all with E.I. Then we share our discovery of dyslexic heart (which is associated with many circulatory complaints) and show how simple exercises can correct both these dyslexias in seconds. The next chapter contains testing and correcting schemes that can help end the fatigue, spaceyness, poor balance, poor coordination, and memory problems in the E.I. Along with the integration exercises, they represent the core of the *physicist's rapid solution*. Then you will find our chapter on ecological nutrition. Here for the first time, nutritional breakthroughs are presented along with possible, ecological conflicts. The reader can then gauge what is in his or her best interests, always with the benefit of MBT. Included here are amino acids, new forms of B-vitamins for the E.I., fatty acids and novel eating tips.

The next two chapters had to be included as this is the first ecological/nutritional book written by a physicist. The reader must see how easy it is for a scientist to prove that the accepted medical methods in the West are anything but scientific! And how our entire (addicted) society suffers because its medical community, in its self-serving interests, continues to deny that ecological *and* energy imbalance are the key factors despite the facts. You will learn true scientific arguments to enable you to judge both medical and complementary health methods. Some modern medical nightmares, all performed under the guise of Science, are demonstrated. The following chapter on Psychology will demonstrate that most mental ills are either ecological or energy blocks. Phobias are revealed to be acupuncture meridian blocks! Rapid, sure-fire corrections for phobias, emotional stress, and psychological reversal (all with MBT) are given. The fallacies and nightmares of modern psychiatry are indicated here. Finally, we close with the practical and a chapter on some fascinating new discoveries of ours that can help many sufferers of E.I. The time of day that you eat something and external weather conditions can determine if you will react to your food! Our Appendices offer additional support. App. A tells you how to reach us or our headquarters in the U.S. and Europe. App. B lists definitive diagnostic tests and App. C lists food families. All footnote references are placed in App. D.

Here are some hints at how to use this book. Throughout, we use **BOLDFACE** type to denote the first time three things are discussed. These are (1) major subheadings (which will also be found in the table of contents), (2) muscle testing or correcting schemes, and (3) frequent abbreviations. We will use *ITALICS* to denote other important topics when they first come up. The most common abbreviations you have already seen—**HEBS** for HUMAN ECOLOGY BALANCING SCIENCES, **E.I.** for Ecologically Ill or Ecological Illness or Environmental Illness, and **MBT**—our way of denoting what is variously called muscle biofeedback testing (here), muscle testing, muscle response testing, Touch For Health, kinesiology, or Applied Kinesiology. Furthermore, Chapter references are denoted by **Ch.**, Appendices by **App.** and Figures (photos or illustrations) by **Fig.** These last three abbreviations will, of course, be followed by a number or letter reference.

We hope this book represents the beginnings of a Science of Healing. If both energy and ecology are balanced, wellness can be attained by everyone. The methods described are safe, easy, inexpensive, effective and fun to do. In spite of bad genes, tremendous stress, poor diet and life-threatening allergies and Candidiasis, the author is well (for the first time in his life). The reader is invited to join the thousands, around the world, that have gotten well with these methods. To those among the millions with Ecological Illness, if you take the responsibility to balance both your energy and ecology, your time has come!

STEVEN ROCHLITZ
Setauket, New York
October, 1988

1

A PHYSICIST AT DEATH'S DOOR

I had been "reasonably unwell" until my 25th year. My mother's physician had told her not to breast feed her children. As a child I was pale with dark circles under my eyes. I had frequent colds and was given antibiotics. Bloody noses and fatigue were also common complaints. Digestive disorders were my worst and most common problem. From ages 3-11, one type of pain had me doubled over for hours at a time. Repeated doctor's visits and x-rays were diagnosed as "nervous stomach." My tonsils were removed when I was 7. My three brothers were bedwetters. They were fortunate enough to get rashes from cow's milk as infants. I didn't and was kept on it.

Mood swings were part of my behavioral pattern. Every Spring and Summer, extreme malaise and joint pain overcame me. I would get car sick and couldn't ride merry-go-rounds without nausea. My first grade teacher told my mother that I was the most nervous child she had ever seen. The emotional conditions of my mother and older brother made growing up "normal" a difficult proposition and survival itself was frequently problematical. My father's cigarette smoke always sickened me; though the medical experts at the time said this couldn't be. I became shy and withdrawn, a complete opposite of my behavior up to the age of four. As my bloody noses and gastrointestinal pain went undiagnosed and we were poor, my mother told me not to tell the school nurse or teacher when I became ill. I did not argue and learned to suffer in silence and do the best I could.

Yet for all this — or perhaps, to some extent, because of it — I was a great student in school. Years went by without my getting less than 100% on math tests. I was second in the entire school's spelling bee contest. School was a way to get away from my troubled home. My love for Science became the only reinforcement in my life. As I grew older, the nervousness grew into almost constant anxiety with feelings of "impending doom." This made all social interactions difficult for me. I was made worse by being told that it was all "psychological." No one ever told me about hypoglycemia or allergies.

In spite of fatigue and anxiety, I graduated college with an honors degree in Physics and headed to graduate school. I moved from NYC to Long Island's leading university. I was soon plagued with the worst fatigue and malaise of my life and had trouble concentrating. The first Spring and Summer, my throat swelled and was in constant pain. The university's infirmary doctor said it must be psychological and recommended Valium® as "most of the graduate students were on it anyway." The next Spring, I developed full-blown hay fever and realized what was happening the year before. Both the outside allergist I saw and the university's allergist refused to give me allergy shots for reasons of personal greed in their squabble over my payments. Tests revealed I was allergic to dust, mold and most pollens. On my own, I then realized that pollen allergies had caused my severe malaise every Spring and Summer since I was a child. The allergists didn't tell me about food allergies at all!

I obtained my Masters degree and became a Ph.D. Candidate in Physics and taught both graduate and undergraduate courses at two Universities by the age of 23. I became aware of nutrition and felt much better the first year I took nutritional supplements — including brewers yeast. A year later, I found myself fighting for survival!

I began suffering from bladder frequency and burning pain which progressed to stones on two occasions. Large spherical nodules began pushing through my skin in several places. I began to suffer from severe migraines, fainting, amnesia. I couldn't focus my eyes and later the fluid in my eyes began gelling up and impinging on my retina. I was getting extreme intestinal pain and was passing mucous. Cardiac arrhythmias began and worsened rapidly. I found myself in hospital emergency rooms several times. I had days when my urine turned clear and I urinated away six pounds in one hour. Blood tests showed endocrine abnormalities and that I had lost half of my white blood cells while many of the remaining ones were abnormal or improperly shaped. The physicians at the university and at Nassau County's largest medical center were unable to help me. Some said it was psychological as the throat swelling and Valium® recommendation were in my medical file and it wasn't anything else obvious. Others dismissed me because I didn't have a familiar disease pattern that they could match drugs with. The most knowledgeable physician admitted he didn't know what was happening and told me to "submit yourself to the Rockefeller Institute. You have a new disease pattern and it's worsening rapidly."

The amnesia, migraines, cardiac arrhythmia and bladder condition all deteriorated. I turned white as a ghost and began fainting even from drinking pure water. As a scientist and a human being, I was appalled at the ignorant, unscientific and uncaring nature of all the physicians I saw. My girlfriend left me as she didn't want to be "around at the end." I saw that I couldn't admit myself to a hospital after the absurdities I experienced in emergency rooms and from the chief endocrinologist and gastroenterologist at the Nassau facility.

It was 1976, and I was vaguely aware that the tall ships were sailing only 50 miles away in New York Harbor while my "boat" was rapidly sinking. I was determined to find the cause myself or die trying—I was in too much pain to want to go on like that much longer. Armed only with the knowledge of what Science is, I began to study medicine in a desperate manner at the university's medical library. I appeared ghost-like and semiconscious. I couldn't function there for too long and I didn't believe I would last long enough to find the answer. I said good-bye to my parents.

After rummaging through urology, nephrology, gastroenterology, endocrinology, immunology and cardiology; I picked up a hematology text. It indicated my blood abnormalities could be cancer, systemic toxicities or systemic allergies. With the nodules appearing on my body, I thought it must be cancer. The county toxicologist said there were no toxins in my urine. While waiting for an allergist's appointment at the Nassau facility's clinic, I found a text first written by Albert Rowe, M.D. in the 1930's. It detailed how food allergies can affect every organ. My set of "unexplainable, new or psychological" symptoms were all there! I decided to fast and got some relief for the first time. Skin allergy tests actually confirmed marked allergy to many foods.

My mother died at this time of pancreatitis at the age of fifty. She never drank alcohol — the physicians' only "explanation". The day before her month long coma began, an attending physician could only diagnose her complaints as "psychological" and gave her a Valium® injection (as her pancreas was exploding). I began receiving allergy shots and soon after I started losing sensation in my arms and legs. Two neurologists said I might be coming down with Multiple Sclerosis. (They said it was too early to tell; but I should "walk back in when I couldn't walk back in.") I had bad reactions to all the allergist's drugs (for allergy and cardiac symptoms, etc.). After several unfortunate years with allergists, I eliminated the shots (which contained phenol) and wheat and dairy (which did not show up on any allergy tests done). Normal sensation returned to me.

Then I became aware of a new medical specialty — Clinical Ecology. I studied this new literature and went to a clinical ecologist. I proved to be a "universal reactor" — sensitive to foods, chemicals and pollens. I had "Twentieth Century Disease" and this "new" condition, Candidiasis. But the drug Nystatin did nothing for me. I was told to coat my walls, phone, etc. with aluminum foil and avoid the twentieth century. Somehow I knew this was no answer. I began studying alternative health modalities. Hypnosis, acupuncture and cranial adjustments helped me, but I was still a universal reactor. I learned to do my own acupuncture.

Then I became aware of Kinesiology (also called Touch For Health and muscle testing and balancing). At a seminar in 1983, I learned of a previously developed method of "asking the body questions" or balancing the body's energies for a specific problem. The brain records everything that has happened to it and the muscle testing is just a biofeedback system to get at this knowledge.

At the class I was reacting to cologne, nail polish remover, etc. As usual, I kept my misery to myself. But I made the bold assumption that I might be able to devise a "Candida Balance" using this new method. I had myself balanced, not stating what I was being balanced for. To my surprise and great discomfort, my face turned red (for a few seconds — a healing reaction) and I felt as if I were burning up! This "balance" took less than an hour to be performed. When I got off the table, I was surprised when I could hardly even smell the cologne that the one fellow always wore and which had previously sickened me. It didn't bother me! I drove home and for the first time in my life, car fumes didn't affect me! Once home, I went to stores and opened paint cans, perfume bottles, etc. with no effect! I began eating foods that previously had made me ill. I ate alfalfa sprouts (a grass) which had caused immediate diarrhea before. Now I was fine. Since alfalfa is a grass, I reasoned that my pollen allergies might now also be gone. Months later when tree and grass pollens appeared, I had no reactions. For the first time in my life, I didn't experience fatigue and malaise in the Spring and Summer. For the first time, I felt well and knew that I had found the tool to remain well.

I wanted to see if I could duplicate this remarkable change on others with Ecological Illness (E.I.). By this time and after years of studying alternative health and nutrition, I had become a holistic health consultant or nutritionist using kinesiology. Within a week (of my balance), I had my first opportunity. Ellen had been ill for eight years. She had been to many physicians with complaints of fatigue, dizziness, malaise, hypoglycemia, dermatitis and more. She was found to be a universal (food, chemical and pollen) reactor on her previous visit. She had trouble even walking on that occasion as her knees gave out, supposedly from adrenal exhaustion. She was also allergic to all the supplements she had been given.

After a two hour balance, she felt much better. Later that day, she was able to eat everything without symptoms! Pollen and chemical allergies met with the same fate. Thus the Candida Balance was born in 1983. Ellen has never needed to repeat the balance. Others that followed did not always have such an immediate effect or last as long as Ellen's balance did. But virtually everyone experiences an immediate improvement in energy, mood, coordination, circulation, overall health and allergy reduction. Those that were tested (like myself) showed that they had overcome immune deficiency – these blood test results would be accepted by any physician. As we shall see, many myths about E.I. were exploded by this work. Eliminating yeast overgrowths and avoiding the 20th Century often do *not* get people with E.I. well.

A year later, I was urged to teach a seminar, so others could perform these methods. Thus in 1984, the Human Ecology Balancing Sciences Seminar was begun. I have taught the H.E.B.S. (or just HEBS) seminar across the U.S., Canada, Europe, Australia and New Zealand to both physicians and "laymen." Now you can begin to learn how ecology and energy balancing, together, are so effective in restoring wellness.

2

ALLERGIES & THE IMMUNE SYSTEM

We begin here with a discussion on the underlying nature of allergies. The many facets of this seemingly complex subject will be unraveled so that everyone can understand it. If you find this chapter difficult — you shouldn't — you can skip it for now and come back later. Please try not to shortchange yourself. One of the many innovations in this book is our discovery that many with allergies have learning blocks and phobias. Do not quit if you find a big, new word here and there! Later chapters contain *rapid, fun corrections* for any learning problems (big words, new words or concepts) that you may have.

First, we need to define our use of the term "allergy." History will guide us here. At the turn of the century, Clemons von Pirquet, M.D., first used "allergy" to mesh the words "altered reactivity." He found that mice promptly died upon receiving the *second* injection of egg protein. Here a higher organism was *reacting* in an *altered* or unusual (and very disastrous) manner to an environmental substance — a food. During the first half of this century, the internal substances responsible for similar reactions in man were discovered. And we will discuss them in this chapter. These substances were then declared by the new medical specialists to be responsible for all allergy. Unfortunately, many allergists declared that if these substances weren't involved in a "reaction," it couldn't be an allergic reaction. Those who insisted that they were allergic to a food, chemical or anything, for that matter, were told "it must be mental" if the allergic substances weren't found.

Most allergists were thus content to treat hives, hay fever, asthma and anaphylaxis—a rapid, life-threatening reaction as in the mice above. Because the substances or mechanisms were different or unknown, most allergists ignored evidence that fatigue, headaches, gastrointestinal disorders, arthritis and many "emotional" disorders were also due to altered reactivity. Allergists who spoke up were chagrinned by their colleagues! Yet the medical literature has always contained such evidence. In fact, ancient Greek physicians often took their patients off milk, and failing this, all food until they got well—regardless of the complaint! The ancient Chinese, Hebrews and others were also aware of food allergy in some form. Recently allergy awareness has had a resurgence. Some would say that allergy has become an epidemic. In the 1930's, leading allergist, Albert Rowe, M.D., said that in civilized society, allergy was second only to infection[1] in the etiology (causation) of disease. Recently, Richard Mackarness, M.D. states that allergy is now the prime cause of most medical complaints.[2]

Here we will revert to the original notion of allergy as any altered reactivity. Any harmful effect on the body, brought about by a food, chemical, pollen or energy (such as microwaves, T.V., etc.) will be called allergy here. We refer to individual responses. If everyone gets sick from something, it would be called a toxicity. Thus, in the spirit of the ancient Greek physicians and the nascent Western medical specialty known as Clinical or Human Ecology or Environmental Medicine, *any* allergy can induce *any* symptom in a given individual.

Ideally, these physicians, instead of relying solely on (allergic) drugs for allergic people—as traditional allergists would—recommend environmental, diet and life-style changes and nutritional supplementation. They may address some of the causes of allergies: weak immune systems, Candidiasis, Parasitosis, etc.

It is crucial, before we see what allergy is, to examine what it isn't. In this post-Freudian age, many have been led to believe that allergies are "all in the mind." Until 25 years ago, allergic hives was called "psychodermatitis." Allergic edema (swelling) was called "angio*neurotic* edema." One can still read medical journals on "psychosomatic medicine" and "see" how asthma and other allergic disorders are caused purely by "emotional stress." If this were true, the whole society would be wheezing.

It is easy to fall into the psychosomatic trap because allergies commonly affect the nervous and endocrine systems and hence the emotions. Historically, the causative role of allergy in ailments of the skin, sinuses, lungs and gastrointestinal tract was very slowly acknowledged by "modern" Western medicine. Allergists have often written of allergy as the "bastard" of medicine. Now the last organ, so desperately in need of recognition of its vulnerability to allergy, is the brain. Unfortunately, many in medicine and psychiatry don't (or won't) accept that emotions and behavior are governed by an all-too-susceptible brain.

If you believe *only* that an illness is "psychological," you will always *appear* to find the psychological causes! The following examples, extracted from the clinical ecology literature will demonstrate this self-fulfilling prophecy.

A nun was beginning to feel depressed. She doubled her efforts in seeking guidance from God, as she believed this was a spiritual problem. Every day she'd light a candle, kneel and pray for God to show her some sign regarding her malady. Soon after, her depression would begin or intensify. To her and her priests, this meant she had sinned and was to be punished. After a long while, she saw an ecologist whose testing revealed she was allergic to the hydrocarbons released from a lit candle! No candles — no depression!

Another example is of a woman executive who would get migraines every Saturday and Sunday. A trail of psychologists and psychiatrists, over the years and with expensive therapy including psychoactive drugs, concluded that guilt from not working on weekends was the cause. Finally, an ecologist's tests revealed she was allergic to the fish she ate every Friday night. No fish—no migraines. In fact, her "Type A" workaholic behavior itself changed when her biochemistry corrected after an allergy elimination diet. Therefore, ecology should be the first (and psychology—the last) factor to look at, for most complaints.

What maladies can allergy cause or be associated with? The following is a partial list. Be aware that the Candidiasis (Parasitosis) list is similar as the two are deeply intertwined. There may also be many other possible causes for many of these complaints. The skilled practitioner makes use of a lengthy history, physical exam and appropriate tests to pin down the cause(s) of an illness.

POSSIBLE ALLERGY SYMPTOMS

Fatigue, dizziness, confusion, headache, migraines, narcolepsy (much of the fatigue syndrome may be a type of sleepiness—narcolepsy would be the extreme), neck ache, backache, arthritis, gastrointestinal(**GI**): gas, pain, bloating, diarrhea, constipation, esophagitis, colitis, ileitis, hemorrhoids, mouth sores, ulcers, indigestion, repeating a taste, muscle aches and twitches (muscles around your eyes twitch?), double vision, hypoglycemia, high blood sugar (diabetes), rashes, hives and other skin disorders, dermographia (skin turns red or white after slight pressure), dyslexia, hyperactivity, bladder frequency, bed wetting, pain on urination, *emotional*: depression, anxiety, paranoia, schizophrenia, cardiac arrhythmias, rapid heart beat, joint swelling, sinusitis, nose runs after eating, shiners under the eyes, earaches, pancreatitis, gallbladder-type pain, high or low blood pressure, anaphylaxis, various abnormal neurological sensations (we like to ask if the subject ever gets an itch that feels like a bug is crawling on the skin?), hot flashes, morning sickness in pregnancy, insomnia, under- and overweight and Candidiasis —yes Candidiasis (or Parasitosis) may somewhat be induced by, as well as itself causing, allergies. And more...

When physicians ask how allergy can cause so much chronic, degenerative illness, we are amazed. After all, if allergy can cause something as "mild" as hay fever and something as extreme as anaphylactic shock (and death), isn't it logical to assume that chronic, degenerative illness which lies between these two extremes can be allergy-induced?! Or would they have us believe that "drug deficiencies" cause all illness?

In explaining how the above complaints can result from some form of allergic reaction, we'll start with a brief review of the immune system and classical allergy. Below is a summary of the immune system's components.

THE IMMUNE SYSTEM

1. Cells
  1A. T-cells with their many subtypes
  1B. B-cells with their many subtypes
2. Immunoglobulins — large protein molecules (not cells)
  2A. Different classes including IgA, IgD, IgE, IgG, IgM. Each has subtypes.

In simple terms, the *IMMUNE SYSTEM* has two types of components. The first is the white blood cell. These cells are further divided into two basic groups: the T-cells (T is for Thymus) and the B-Cells (B is for bone marrow.) These names were derived from the presumed manufacturing sites of the respective cells. These cells are again subdivided. E.g., T-cells are classified as T-helper, T-killer, T-suppressor, etc. These names are based on the functions of these respective cells. Once again, each of these last cells are further subdivided, but we needn't delve into this.

The B-Cells manufacture the second major type of immune system component — the *IMMUNOGLOBULINS*. These are not cells; the big word is easily understood. It simply means a large, spherical (or globular), protein molecule of the immune system. Its abbreviation is Ig, pronounced I-Gee. There are several types of immunoglobulins, namely IgA, IgD, IgE, IgG, IgM. And these are further subdivided; which we needn't go into again. The immunoglobulin is made by the B-cells in response to the presence of a foreign protein (or protein-like) substance in the blood. The immunoglobulin is also called the humoral (blood) antibody and the foreign substance is called the *antigen* or *allergen* (if an allergic reaction is involved). The classical allergic reaction is also called the *ANTIBODY-ANTIGEN REACTION*.

The classic, allergic symptoms noted earlier often involve a reaction of relatively large amounts of IgE. This is how the allergist *defines* allergy. Some allergists are finally examining allergic reactions due to other antibodies, e.g. IgG. All the

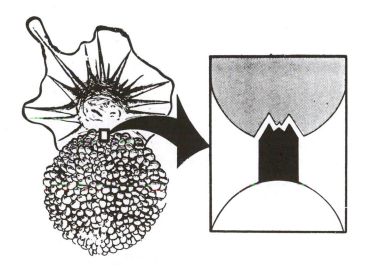

Figure 1.

The lock-and-key analogy of the antibody-antigen reaction. *Left*: An antibody latching on to the protein markers. *Right*: the lock-and-key close-up.

immunoglobulins are capable of forming antibody-antigen complexes in the lock-and-key analogy depicted in Fig. 1.

There can be a sharp distinction between classical allergy and some clinical ecologists' models of allergy. Instead of involving high IgE, immunodeficiency may be responsible for some allergy. Many with multiple allergies and Candidiasis are severely deficient in either or both cellular and protein antibody components of the immune system.

This brings us to one possible cause of chronic allergy — low IgA. IgA was meant to coat the body's mucous membranes found in the sinuses, respiratory tract, under the skin, in the gastrointestinal tract, vagina, etc. It is called (s)IgA. The "s" is for secretory. (s)IgA serves as a barrier to the external world. It is meant to keep undigested food molecules from being absorbed into the blood from the gastrointestinal (GI) tract mucosa and to keep airborne chemicals and pollens and germs from being absorbed through the skin, sinuses, lungs, etc.

Undigested food can cause great harm if it enters the blood through the GI mucosa. Likewise for foreign substances entering through the other mucous membranes, if (s)IgA is low. Two kinds of reactions can occur. The first is immunological, namely the production of antibodies which would then react with the foreign substance; now the antigen or allergen. You see, the primary purpose of the immune system is to recognize and destroy germs or anything foreign to the body. Bacteria, viruses, etc. have protein molecules which stick out of their cell membranes or walls. See the left side in Fig. 1. These act as markers; indeed our own cells have their own markers. These markers are what the immune system components look for in deciding what is "of the body" and what is foreign. The foreign markers also serve as templates in the rapid production of antibodies should a germ be found in the body. The lock-and-key mechanism is again involved in this production. Immune components attach to the foreign markers and make a master key.

Now the immune system can't distinguish food "markers"

from an invading germ. Thus if an undigested food (especially protein) molecule enters the blood (see Fig. 2), large amounts of antibodies may be made. An allergic reaction may ensue. This, you recall, is how allergy was discovered. The first injection of egg protein into the animal's blood — bypassing the IgA (and other) protection — led to the creation of antibodies. These were present to react to the second injection of protein. The substances released from the resulting antibody-antigen reaction were of sufficient amount and toxicity to promptly kill the mouse. Later we will discuss the second type of reaction; this involves a direct effect on the body's tissues by the undigested substance.

First, let's examine the substances, or *mediators*, released by the allergic reaction. The first is the well known histamine. It can cause smooth muscle contraction. These muscles are controlled by the autonomic nervous system, unlike the skeletal motions which we readily control for motion. Smooth muscles control breathing and GI functions, etc. It is also a potent

Figure 2. Normal (top) and too-permeable (bottom) gastrointestinal mucosae.

Top: Only single amino acids get through the mucosa and into the blood.

Bottom: Unbroken-down peptides (3 amino acids) are absorbed.

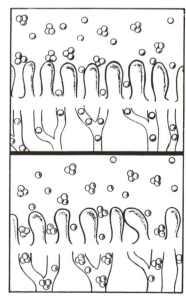

vasoactive substance, i.e. it can dilate the blood vessels. If the vessels in your nose dilate, they may "leak" and your nose runs. Thus hay fever symptoms can occur. Capillary permeability is said to be increased. It was first thought that histamine receptors existed only on skin, sinus, respiratory tissues and blood vessels. (If a cell has histamine *receptors* on its membrane, it will absorb, and thus be affected, by histamine. The lock-and-key mechanism is again at work here.) More recently, a different type of histamine receptor—H_2—was found in GI and brain tissue.

SUBSTANCES CREATED AFTER AN ALLERGIC REACTION

1. Histamine
2. Serotonin
3. SRS-A or Leukotriene (pronounced lew-ko-try-een)
4. Kinins
5. Prostaglandins
6. Complement
7. Immune complexes

One organ in the brain replete with H_2 receptors is the hypothalamus.[3] Its many functions include controlling appetite, sleep, emotions and the pituitary gland. The last was formerly known as the "master" of the endocrine system. The hypothalamus is also near a region of the brain which is not well protected by the usual blood-brain barrier. The latter allows only glucose and a few other simple substances to enter the brain. So from this one mechanism, histamine from an allergic reaction is capable of affecting emotions, energy-level, sleep pattern, appetite, weight and the endocrine system. There is, in part, a genetic predisposition regarding which organs have histamine receptors as well as the amounts present. But this can change with life experience. Headaches can be caused by histamine in two ways. One is a simple clogging of the sinuses, such as in the temple area. Such headaches are often called tension headaches until allergy is investigated. Secondly, histamine or other allergic mediators can dilate blood vessels; pain results as this stretching affects the nerves that run along blood vessels. The brain itself may swell ever so slightly. This is called cerebral edema and this can cause any neurological or "emotional" symptom. If major blood vessels (such as those near the heart) are dilated from a large amount of histamine or similar mediator, the blood pressure may drop to zero and death can result. This is part of the anaphylactic reaction such as from the second penicillin injection that you may have heard of.

Now what does the presence of histamine receptors in GI tissue tell us? It implies that much of GI illness is caused by, or related to, allergy. This includes ulcers, colitis, etc. Let's look at ulcers. Once the most widely prescribed drug in America was Tagamet®. (It replaced Valium® years ago as #1.) The Physician's Desk Reference states that Tagamet® is an "H_2 antagonist."[4] This means Tagamet® binds to the stomach's mast cells and prevents them from absorbing histamine. If histamine is absorbed, it triggers a large acid outpour which can lead to an ulcer. But why is there histamine in the stomach in the first place? Yes, food allergy is the likely answer. Clearly, a preferential treatment would be ascertaining and eliminating allergies! Tagamet®, once thought to be free of side effects, is now known to have many; this includes a possible role in Candidiasis. The role of allergy in colitis and ileitis was proven 50 years ago. Yet even today, GI specialists hypothesize mythical viruses and pump their patients with drugs that don't get at the cause of the problem. Allergy gets swept under the rug, at the patient's expense, once again.

Let's examine another GI complaint not discussed in similar books. It's called *dumping syndrome* and refers to the spasming of the pyloric valve (between the stomach and the small intestine). If this valve opens too much, the stomach's contents will enter the small intestine too quickly. If a large amount of food or even water enters, a large amount of blood will pool there to hypothetically absorb nutrients. There will then be a sudden lack of blood for the rest of the body, especially the brain. A hypovolemic, or low blood volume, reaction occurs. The person may then faint. This happened to the author on numerous occasions and was undiagnosed by physicians (but was in Rowe's text). Some "Universal Reactors" may not really be; rather pylorospasm or dumping syndrome could cause symptoms after eating *anything*. This appears to be unknown to most in the ecology field.

Now, another substance released by an allergic reaction is serotonin. Like histamine, which it closely resembles, it is a neurotransmitter. This type of chemical is responsible for how we think and feel and for the transmission of signals along the entire nervous system. Low serotonin can cause depression, obsessive-compulsive behavior and insomnia. Apparently the circadian (24-hour cycle) rhythm is affected by serotonin or other allergic mediators. High levels of serotonin may cause asthma or sinusitis. Exposure to negative ions can normalize serotonin levels. Do you feel better in the shower or at a water-fall or near a man-made negative ion generator?

Another allergic mediator was first called SRS-A or Slow Reacting Substance of Anaphylaxis. It's now called a leukotriene (pronounced lew-ko-try-een). It can cause asthma and anaphylactic reactions. It is vasoactive and can cause smooth muscle contraction, like histamine. Another class of allergic mediator is the kinin. It is a smooth muscle contractor. This inflammatory substance may cause aches, swelling and pains in muscles, joints, sinuses, etc. Kinins may also be a secondary mediator. Here it would not be released from the allergic reaction, but it would be released as a response to the primary mediators. Another secondary mediator is prostaglandin. It also causes inflammation. Finally formation of large antibody-antigen complexes and their subsequent complement formation are capable of temporarily clogging up joints, blood vessels, etc. with resultant local trauma.

All these mediators of allergic reactions are vasoactive, inflammatory and/or capable of altering nerve transmission. Thus it should be clear that "allergies can cause any symptom." The many quirks of allergy as an immune reaction are still to be unraveled. We have even observed some people having less reactions when they had a cold. In the first stages of getting a cold, avoiding allergens may prevent the cold. Once the cold exists, some allergens seem to provoke less symptoms! Perhaps the immune system is then more concerned with germs than food particles.

Now let's return to the idea of immunodeficiency, specifically low (s)IgA. Recall that someone with a low amount of this antibody on his mucous membranes is more vulnerable and *PERMEABLE to the external world*. Here, even if no antibody-antigen reaction takes place, the substances entering the blood may directly affect any susceptible organ. Though permeability is a key to understanding **E.I.**, it is not the only answer. (Recall, E.I. refers to Ecological Illness or allergies, Candidiasis and related ills.) Many people have had blood tests reveal undigested proteins in their blood, yet they were not having allergic reactions. Energy imbalance is part of the answer to this anomaly, as we shall see.

Permeability is not the only factor responsible for the allergy "epidemic." Let's list the others now. Many are interrelated. Anything that affects the body's immune or detoxifying organs can be a factor.

FACTORS THAT CAN CAUSE ALLERGY

1. Eating the same foods too often. Likewise for overexposure to pollens, chemicals and even harmful energies.

2. Genetic predisposition. Many families have members with the same allergic response to the same food. (Fortunately, this book will make it clear that you can overcome any allergy.)

3. Candidiasis. Especially if multiple pollen, "universal" food and chemical allergies are present.

4. Other organisms or infections can stress the immune system, such as parasites, viruses, etc. Pets can harbor microorganisms.
5. Hypoglycemia or diabetes. Faulty insulin and blood sugar levels may be caused by allergies, but this probably works the other way around too.
6. Eating toxic, artificial, nutrient-deficient food. Overeating can actually lead to malnutrition too.
7. Specific nutritional deficiencies especially the anti-oxidants needed by the immune system.
8. Chemical and electromagnetic smog and radiation.
9. Heavy metal toxicity such as mercury.
10. Fluoride weakens the immune system.
11. Lack of breast feeding of infants. Nutrients and protective antibodies not found in any "formula" exist in mother's milk. An entire generation has suffered because they did not receive mother's milk because Western pediatricians, under the false guise of science discouraged it!
12. Emotional stress and the poor handling of it in our society.
13. Lack of exercise.
14. Improper structural alignment, especially in the cranium and jaw (TMJ or temporomandibular joint).
15. Endocrine disorders.

All these things can lead to an immune system breakdown. Allergies, autoimmune disease (like lupus), cancer or immunodeficiency can result. At least it appears that most with universal allergies do not get cancer. And again when the underlying factors are identified and eliminated or balanced, most allergies can be eradicated.

3

HYPOGLYCEMIA & DIABETES – THE ALLERGY CONNECTION

Perhaps the first (often undiagnosed) allergic symptom for many people is faulty blood sugar. William Philpott, M.D., and his biochemist collaborators, have found that the **PANCREAS** is often directly affected[5] by undigested proteins and fats. Such an organ is called a *shock organ*. Different undigested foods may preferentially attack different organs or tissues. Gluten, especially wheat gluten, can affect the GI tract, nervous system and liver. Philpott has found elevated liver enzymes in some people as a response to eating wheat. Tomatoes and other nightshades (potato, peppers, tobacco) have recently been re-discovered to cause arthritic symptoms. Tomatoes contain a relatively high amount of toxic alkaloids and were avoided by man until the last 100 years or so. (This coincides with the present, self-serving Psychiatric Age. People used to be as intelligent as lower animals who will avoid, *for the rest of their lives*, any food that adversely affects them. Now people have been brainwashed to believe chronic or episodic complaints are due to drug deficiencies or couch-lying deficiencies.)

Philpott's books link allergies with hypoglycemia and diabetes[6] by viewing the pancreas as a shock organ. He performed clinical tests which proved that individual allergic-type responses to foods and chemicals can cause low and high blood sugar reactions. Fasting glucose and insulin levels were taken of people in an ecological setting. These tests were repeated after ingestion or inhalation of potential allergens. These foods, etc. need not contain sugar or carbohydrates! Yet blood sugar levels can change dramatically. Most people, apparently have a rise in blood sugar. This includes the so-called hypoglycemic. The latter, under fasting conditions is thus revealed to be a type of diabetic. Philpott uses the term "chemical diabetes" to signify high blood sugar reactions to individual foods. So most hypoglycemics are really chemical diabetics. This isn't surprising, as many in holistic health know the scenario of the skinny, nervous hypoglycemic who eventually becomes the overweight, fatigued "maturity onset" diabetic.

Now the medical orthodoxy still denies the existence of hypoglycemia. And many holistic practitioners recommend low carbohydrate and high protein diets. Yet, when tested individually, the "hypoglycemic" may tolerate maple syrup and not tolerate a protein food like beef or cheese. And these latter foods may well affect the blood sugar! Hypoglycemia's possible symptoms are listed below.

HALLMARKS OF HYPOGLYCEMIA
1. Fatigue
2. Spaceyness, giddiness, mental confusion
3. Sleepiness
4. Frequent hunger pains, even shortly after eating
5. Anxiety, nervous overreactivity, trepidations, insecurity, panic attacks, phobias
6. Depression
7. Muscle cramps (Can also be caused by an allergic, over-acid condition and lack of oxygenation of the muscles)
8. Eye symptoms: Inability to focus eyes (convergence insufficiency), seeing spots

Let's see how these complaints come about. When the blood

sugars change significantly, the entire endocrine system may be alerted. This system has been likened to an orchestra, always attempting to maintain (chemical) harmony. Dropping blood sugar levels alert the adrenals to secrete its hormones. These include adrenalin and other stress hormones. But while running on adrenalin (instead of a steady glucose level) may prevent fainting—it can be a nightmarish existence. The excess adrenal hormones or fluctuating blood sugar and insulin levels often coincide with anxiety, trepidations, feelings of impending doom, dizziness, sleepiness, confusion, insecurity, fatigue, frequent hunger pangs, and depression. Even autism, this researcher has found is due to severe blood sugar reactions, allergies and ultimately parasitosis. Recently, medical researchers have found that a protein in cow's milk destroys the insulin-producing cells of the pancreas!

Mid-afternoon is often when the hypoglycemic will be overcome with fatigue or sleepiness. This author has found that corn induces hypoglycemia in many people. (This may relate to an unusual ratio of the amino acids leucine and isoleucine in corn. Or corn may induce hypoglycemia because of its high mold content from being stored. The mold poison, aflatoxin is found in corn ([and peanut] products.) In Mexico, where corn is the main staple, what time do the people take their siesta? Yes, it's mid-afternoon. It is fascinating to see how different societies counteract their hypoglycemia in diverse ways. In Britain, tea (caffeine) time is also 3-4 P.M. Returning to corn, it may be fortunate that the sugar used for blood sugar tests is dextrose. This is derived from corn. (If you are allergic to a food, you may well react to anything that is derived from it.) It is impossible to remove 100% of the protein antigens that the derivative comes from. Most allergists think of sucrose, the commonest sugar, as incapable of causing allergic reactions. But there will always be some cane or beet antigens (from which the sugar was derived) left behind—as well as processing chemicals. Sucrose may also be involved with Candidiasis; in disguised form, it may find its way onto your table. E.g., caramel is really burnt sugar. Maple syrup may be less allergenic than sucrose, dextrose or honey.

Many people are now being tested for hypoglycemia by an

orthodox physician. This is a grave error. Some people, during the test, fall asleep, pass out, get convulsions, "the shakes," or strange emotional reactions. But the physician has memorized a number in medical school that is "the threshold" for hypoglycemia. If the patient's levels don't fall below this level, he is told he has normal sugar metabolism?! What he may have experienced during the test is irrelevant. The truth is that the *rate* of change of the blood sugar level is at least as important as the actual level. Rising or falling rapidly can cause any of the above symptoms, regardless of the actual level reached.

Fig. 3 shows a graph with a normal blood sugar, and several variants of abnormal blood sugar ranges. The normal graph (A) depicts a slow rise (after drinking the sugar solution after a 12 hour fast), long leveling off and slow decline. Graph B is classical hypoglycemia — a drop below 50. But graph D is also hypoglycemic — note the rapid rise and rapid decline — even though 50 is not reached. Graph C is a diabetic reaction — high blood sugar. Perhaps if the patient were fasting long enough, or

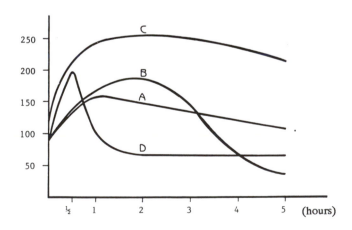

Figure 3.

Normal (A) and abnormal (B,C,D) blood sugar graphs.

avoided corn for five days, graphs B or D would look like C, as indicated by Philpott. Always remember that your own symptoms may be the most definitive gauge of faulty blood sugar reactions. Thus you can test yourself, obviating blood tests—if you don't suspect a severe problem.

DIABETICS can also attain great benefit from complete allergy testing. Philpott has written of the allergy connection to both juvenile and maturity-onset diabetes. The nature and amount of carbohydrate in a food may be of much less importance to the diabetic's insulin requirements than the allergenicity of the food. It is shocking that "diabetologists" don't even test for allergy to the insulin that their patients are taking. This is a common problem! Insulin sources were beef, pork, or beef and pork. Now there is the so-called genetically engineered, or human insulin. Bacteria are the actual manufacturers of this insulin. There are, of course, excipients in all injectables and there are slow releasing or lente forms. The diabetic, can often greatly reduce insulin requirements by eliminating allergenic insulin! Avoiding allergic foods and receiving other pancreas support—including digestive enzymes and bicarbonates—provide further benefit to the diabetic. Along with all the other modalities in this book, it is easy to have most maturity diabetics off insulin. And the juvenile diabetics can usually eliminate ⅔ of their insulin requirements. (Nutrients needed include chromium, amino acids, zinc; and energy balancing is just as crucial.)

This researcher also believes that hypoglycemic and diabetic reactions may also be induced by a Parasitosis-potassium defect or by Candidiasis or by the die-off involved.

Let's return to digestion. When enough digestive enzymes were given before a meal, Philpott found that absorption of undigested foods could be precluded. If the stomach needs assistance, a supplement of pepsin and betaine hydrochloride can be given. Parasitosis often leads to low levels of stomach acid and pepsin. Many people, as they age, have a diminished stomach acidity. Their food is not properly digested. The resultant pain, discomfort or gas leads them to take antacids — the opposite of what they really need to get at the cause of the problem. In addition to pepsin and acid supplements with the meal, bicarbonates may be recommended 45 minutes *after* eating to alkalinize the intestines and counteract the acidosis (acid state) that may ensue from an allergic reaction.

Let's look at the pancreas as a shock organ. This shock organ may be involved in a *VICIOUS CYCLE*. The pancreas, in addition to producing insulin and other hormones, secretes digestive enzymes. These include pancreatin and alkaline salts (bicarbonates) that go to the small intestine. While the stomach needs to be acid (to break down proteins and destroy germs), the intestines need to be alkaline. In fact stomach acidity triggers the pancreas to make the small intestine alkaline. So paradoxically, if the stomach is not acid enough, the intestines will be too acid. Undigested proteins or fats from a *too*-permeable, gastrointestinal mucosa can enter the blood and travel to, and be absorbed by, the pancreas. It may be shocked into doing several harmful things. It may over- or under-produce insulin resulting in hypoglycemia (low blood sugar) and diabetes, respectively. Or it may under-produce the digestive enzymes; but the unavailability of these makes it likely that undigested food molecules will be absorbed in the GI tract. *This is the vicious cycle.* It can be halted by an allergy-elimination diet and/or digestive enzyme supplementation.

By the way, the connection between allergies and poor digestion allows for *SEVERAL "FREE" TYPES OF "ALLERGY TESTS"*. If undigested food appears in your stool or you can smell undigested food molecules in your urine, you should avoid those foods. (Another unrelated, but "free" test is the Coca pulse test. If your pulse rate changes within an hour of eating something, an allergy probably exists. This test will miss some food allergies.)

The pancreas is not the only shock organ of allergic reactions or undigested foods. The liver, spleen, lymph system, nervous system, endocrine glands, joints, kidneys and the GI tract may be directly affected. Some medical researchers claim that most foods contain some harmful ingredients; "minimal" eating is recommended.[7] We have already noted the alkaloids in tomatoes and other nightshades. Nicotine and caffeine are also potent alkaloids. Soon we will discuss exorphins found in grains, milk and legumes. Virtually all plants contain a class of proteins called lectins. These are suspect in some cases of celiac disease, arthritis, kidney and immune disorders. Seeds, grains, legumes and tubers (root vegetables) contain high amounts of lectins which may not be broken down by cooking. Many foods also contain anti-vitamin, anti-mineral, anti-enzyme, hormone-like, toxic or carcinogenic substances. And agricultural technicians now create new hybrid grains that can be foreign to our systems. Our primitive ancestors probably didn't have the opportunity to overeat as we do; finding pleasures other than eating seems prudent. We don't wish to cause alarm, but the old adage warns that we should "eat to live and not live to eat." *Small portions of food may be the way we were meant to eat.* Allergies and hypoglycemia may be minimized in this way too.

Never forget, too, that hypoglycemia is nothing but a symptom of deeper problems — allergies, Candidiasis, etc. There are many health books published each year that look at hypoglycemia or allergies or Candida or Epstein-Barr Syndrome from an (unfortunately) isolated point of view. None of them has any real solution either — though they always offer some "magic" pill. By the end of this book, you'll know why that will never work! This author — a physicist — has united them all, for the first time. Physicists are trained to unite (seemingly) separate forces of nature and to be honest about a *real* solution!

4

FOOD ADDICTION, ALLERGIES & ALCOHOLISM

One of the hallmarks of allergy is *ADDICTION* and its accompanying *WITHDRAWAL*. This is the allergy-addiction syndrome whose biochemical origins we will shortly reveal. Any food you crave, or like to eat often, is (or is likely to become) an allergy. Many people don't want to admit their cravings and addictions. Some practitioners automatically denote a food as an allergy-addiction if it's eaten more than three times a week. In nature, there were no refrigerators or kitchen cupboards to allow habitual eating patterns. Nor were most present-day foods, food combinations and amounts available. So your allergies will either be your favorite foods or, conversely, foods you know will make you ill. Foods that you "just don't care for" may be the best for you! They won't get you high as your allergenic foods do. Another clue that allergy may be the cause of a complaint is its *EPISODIC* (comes and goes) nature. An infection or traumatized organ or other possible causes should not manifest with an episodic nature as allergy does, due to the episodic *exposure* to the allergen.

Eating a food everyday without any "obvious" reaction is an example of the *MASKING EFFECT*. I.e., the worst symptoms are masked as the body attempts to adapt to the stress. Masking and allergy-addiction can also occur for chemicals, pollens etc. It can be shocking to find out your favorite foods are your worst allergies. But this is one of the causes of allergy. It's no coincidence that the most frequently eaten foods in our society are also the most common allergies. This includes wheat, corn, sugar, coffee, milk, peanuts, chocolate, eggs, oranges, tobacco, tomatoes, beef and yeast. One eats the foods one is allergic to everyday precisely to avoid the effects of withdrawal. Food addiction withdrawal can be as nightmarish as drug addiction withdrawal. One clinical ecologist recalls a woman patient begging him to kill her because she couldn't handle the withdrawal. Headache, fatigue, depression, arthritis and other symptoms are common. Food withdrawal lasts from 4-12 days, typically about 5 days. Chemical withdrawal can last up to 3 weeks.

Many people eat only 5-10 foods; going from one allergy-addiction to the next. We are an addicted society! (Many will not admit to having "cravings," so "likes" may have to be the term you think of.) The 24-hour convenience stores know about cravings and only stock foods that people will need a "fix" for. You won't find codfish there. In HEBS we call these stores, "allergy-addiction headquarters." One addiction begets another. The cigarette smoker and coffee drinker are probably allergic to these items, which also induce hypoglycemia. Decaffeinated beverages are a myth as they still contain 3% caffeine and many other toxins or allergens and the caffeine itself can still be a severe allergy at the 3%!

Giving up all allergenic and hypoglycemia-inducing substances at the same time is the best way to go. Don't try giving up a different allergy/addiction each week. You'll go through continuous misery and probably won't succeed. Don't think of the rest of your life; during that first week, think only of *five* days. At the end of the five days, you'll probably feel better than you have all your life. You'll want to stay on your optimum diet! This book has many tips on preventing or overcoming withdrawal.

Let's return to caffeine and its connection to nicotine. The urge for a cigarette can be due to the caffeine just imbibed or to sugar or to a food in the same family as tobacco (e.g., tomato or potato – see App. C) or to inhaling someone else's smoke. Caffeine, by the way, is found in coffee, tea (except most herb teas), cola, and chocolate. (Chocolate is often easy to give up when you find out it has a high content of roaches and other insects. They can't be kept out of silos, so the amount – several per cent – is regulated.)

With appropriate action now, there doesn't have to be a miserable, lengthy withdrawal for the smoker as these other items were causing some of the withdrawal! Unless you receive the energy balancing, in general, the worse the allergy – the worse the withdrawal.

Let's look more closely at alcoholism. In the 50's, Theron Randolph, M.D. – the father of clinical ecology – showed that alcoholism may not be addiction to alcohol as much as it is addiction to other food derivatives in the beverage.[8] This could be the source of the alcohol; e.g., wheat, rye, potato, rice, grapes or the sugar, yeast, hops, etc. that are added. In the early stages of alcoholism, there is usually a favorite beverage indicating allergy to a substance. The alcoholic thus needs complete allergy testing to avoid foods that are the cause of the "alcoholism." Eating such foods can cause a craving for the alcoholic beverage that contains it. Avoiding these foods may obviate a miserable, lengthy withdrawal. At alcoholics' meetings, most members are eating cakes and drinking coffee (and smoking cigarettes). Thus the underlying allergies, hypoglycemia and Candidiasis are not being addressed. The last two disorders are likely involved if "any beverage will do" for the alcoholic.

We should note that there is a strong connection between alcoholism and societal pressures. We have observed this correlation on our world lecturing tours. It seems that most native peoples, after being displaced by the influx of conquering Caucasians, have a high incidence of alcoholism and other addictions. This is true of the American Indian, the Alaskan Eskimo, the Australian Aborigine, the New Zealand Maori and other native peoples. We have deduced numerous factors that may be responsible for these addictions.

First is the genetic factor. Intermarrying amongst a small population of similar people can lead to a weaker immune system or other metabolic defects. Many world class athletes have been blessed with a mixed set of genes from very *different* races. The opposite can lead to allergies (and addictions) via a weak immune system. Secondly, great emotional stress has surely occurred to these people and their ancestors after being conquered—and sometimes nearly exterminated. Emotional stress can also weaken the immune system and help lead to any malady, including allergy/addiction. The third factor is the rapid, sudden introduction of new foods which were alien to the native people. They may be harmful or allergenic. You know what the paradoxical result may be. Yes, it's addiction!

The fourth factor is simple poverty. This leads to eating nutrient-poor, or so-called junk, food. Addictive mechanisms are then in play. This can then lead to an unfolding of other addictions: cigarettes, alcohol, and sometimes ultimately drugs. A large percentage of addicts are from the ranks of the poor. Crime may then be resorted to, in order to pay for these addictions.[A]

Let's examine the *FOOD FAMILY* concept more closely now. Related plant or animal foods may cross-react as they contain similar or identical proteins or other components. E.g., grains (wheat, rye, barley, corn, oats, rice and millet) are grasses which may be similar to some airborne grass pollens. And all grains except rice and millet have gluten—which can cause GI, and brain symptoms in many. Some food family relationships may surprise you. Poison ivy, cashews and mangoes are in the same family. Note: muscle biofeedback testing (MBT) enables you to determine if all the members of a food family are allergenic. This is often not the case.

The *ROTARY DIVERSIFIED DIET* (**RDD**) is based on the food family concept. If, for example, you are on a 5-day RDD, you will eat the same food only on the fifth day after you last ate it. Also, other foods in the same family would be avoided for two days. The interval of avoidance can vary from 4 days to 2 weeks depending on the severity of the allergies. This diet, though not a cure, can help stabilize the allergic person and prevent new allergies from arising. With a long enough period of avoidance, some foods may again be tolerated on a *rotating basis*. This is because most allergies are said to be cyclical and not fixed. It is important after your allergy testing, that you do not start eating "safe" foods every day as these may become allergenic too. The RDD may help prevent this. It does require discipline to adhere to the RDD concept. But some relaxed form of the RDD is a good idea for most of us.

Let's take a quick look at—one of the most allergic and addictive foods—*dairy products*, now becoming infamous for causing GI and circulatory ills. Simply put, pasteurized, homogenized cow's milk products are among the worst foods man can eat. Don't be fooled by the earlier nutritionists' dogma; it is unnatural for man to consume these milk products! In nature, a mammal ingests *only* its mother's milk and *only* in its infancy. It may take 100,000 years or more to adapt to a food; milk products have only been ingested for a few thousand years. Whether it comes from a machine is not a viable definition of unnatural! The proteins (casein, lactalbumin, whey) found even in raw milk can be allergenic. And most adults are said to eventually develop intolerance to the sugars—lactose and galactose—found in milk. Lactose intolerance can be due to milk allergy. The homogenization and pasteurization process is also said to create the enzyme, xanthine oxidase. In large amounts, this substance is toxic to the blood vessels and initiates cardiovascular illness. Autopsies of 18 year-olds killed in Vietnam revealed the blood vessels of old men. Xanthine oxidase from dairy products is the probable cause. In Europe, raw goat's milk is used with better results. This still contains lactose and molds, though. Commercial dairy products may even be a poor source of calcium. Raw milk contains an enzyme which splits calcium from the phosphorus it's bound to. Pasteurization destroys this enzyme; so humans may not be able to utilize the calcium in milk. And do not trust any nutritional "news" that may have been sponsored by a grant from the dairy industry! Also fat-free milk is usually no less harmful as it still contains allergenic proteins and undigestible sugars. Finally, mother's milk can entail its own risks as the baby may suffer if the mother doesn't avoid foods that she is allergic to. Undigested proteins can enter her milk and affect the infant.

One last thing about milk. Milk is alkaline or basic – the opposite of acidic. Alkalinity counteracts acidity – such as in an ulcerous stomach. This was the rationale for gastroenterologists to put their ulcer patients on a milk diet. Most now know better. Recall that gastric, allergic reactions lead to histamine, and subsequent acid, release. But milk being alkaline can counteract its own acid release – temporarily. Hours later though, an acid or sour stomach can still result. We often say, "show me someone who wakes up with an acid stomach, and I'll show you someone who felt great drinking milk the night before."

Another food, only recently eaten by man is wheat. Some say it is an unnatural hybrid; cultivated and eaten only in the last 5000 years. Anthropologists cite cave drawings depicting arthritis and schizophrenia at times coinciding with the first ingestion of wheat.

Now if a food (like milk) causes GI irritation, its nutrients will not be well absorbed. The irritation can lower absorbability of nutrients from other foods for *days*. Therefore, *the allergenicity of a food takes precedence over its theoretical nutritive value*. The non-absorbability of spinach's iron is analogous to milk's calcium. In spinach, iron is bound to undigestible oxalate (which is capable of causing kidney stones in some people). Chronic

GI irritation from eating allergic foods or from eating too much food is a leading cause of malnutrition in affluent or civilized(?) societies. Undigested food molecules may also be absorbed from GI irritation and result in allergic reactions.

Now the phases of allergy can be shown to fit Hans Selye's *general stress profile.*[9] In the 1930's, Selye found that in "all" illness, there occurred several, identical, physiological changes. Most of his work was done with mice. He called this the General Adaptation Syndrome (**GAS**). In the first stage (the alarm stage), there is a very high adrenal output to counteract the initial stress. The stress, not yet adapted to, is a great shock to the body. If the stress continues, the body *ADAPTS* and this stage may be called the stage of resistance. Here, adrenal output comes down somewhat as the stress is being countered by some body resource. The third stage is called exhaustion as the body's resources are depleted and the adrenals themselves are "running out." The organism is nearing death and the adrenals have shrunk.

Allergy fits into this 3-stage GAS very nicely. Upon initial exposure, the body is shocked and doesn't yet know how to cope except for the adrenal output. Thus an allergen produces an alarm reaction, e.g., the first cigarette anyone smokes causes coughing or nausea. If the individual forces himself to continue smoking, he will adapt and will not react severely each time he smokes. The body has found some resource to cope with the allergens (and toxins). The worst symptoms are masked. If he quits smoking, and then inhales some smoke, he will have an alarm reaction again as he's back in phase 1. Former smokers are among the staunchest anti-smokers, because they were allergic to it all along. Stage three is eventually reached for all habitual smokers and the exhaustion phase is marked by some illness. Adaptation has been overcome.

The body copes well, if forced to, during the adaptation phase. The person may even feel *better* after eating or breathing the allergen, in part because there is an adrenal rush. This phase has its ups and downs. But ingesting a small amount of an allergen or even a larger amount of a food that is only slightly allergic to the body can actually cause a hyper reaction. The person's energy level or mood can be elevated. This may occur for a stage 2 reaction but in the latter case, there will be a downside some time later. Again the downside includes fatigue, depression, etc. A hyperactive child is probably reacting (in stage 1 or 2) to allergens. Long before the term hyperactive was used, allergists described a "tension-fatigue" syndrome in children. The fatigue aspect referred to the fact that some children, after a hyper day, fell dead asleep at an early hour. Manic-depression too is likely the up and down reaction of allergy exposure and withdrawal.

Addictions can, in fact, be a great clue for getting at the under-lying cause of your problems. If you crave sweets, look at hypoglycemia. If you crave sweets and foods containing yeast or mold (see Ch. 7), look for a Candida problem. If you crave foods not in these categories, allergies on their own should be examined. Of course, you may have several of these maladies simultaneously as they are deeply intertwined.

If a person is content to "eat his poison" while in the adaptation phase, he should be aware that at any time, he could enter the final, exhaustion stage. We believe many famous athletes have had this happen, including boxers Mohammed Ali and Jake LaMotta. In their younger days, they were thin with unlimited energy. Overweight and fatigue marked their later days as stage 1 became stage 2 or 3. In fact, in the autobiographical movie of Jake LaMotta, "*RAGING BULL,*" this boxer would irrationally accuse his wife and brother of things they couldn't possibly have done. The movie even showed these fits occurring after eating! Ali, many ecological experts agree, is likely suffering (in part) from allergies or Candidiasis. His mother was very overweight too. The news media has revealed that heavyweight champion, Mike Tyson, has suffered from "manic-depression" all his life. This, most ecologists would agree, is likely the effects of allergy exposure and subsequent withdrawal. Hopefully someone will inform this great boxer, so he won't have to jeopardize his career and waste time with inappropriate "mental therapy". Some great athletes have also suffered from asthma; this too fits in with this discussion on how some types of allergy can actually perk up (physically or mentally) an individual. Other noted personalities were known to get a lift from foods all their lives. Churchill is said to have been perked up from scotch or cigars until his dying day.

Now many health food store remedies or "energizers" may just be producing very mild allergy-alarm reactions. Let's look at the popular bee pollen. It really doesn't contain any magical nutrients unavailable elsewhere. But it does contain traces of pollen and maybe bee proteins. Now many people have slight pollen allergies that they may be unaware of. A small, infrequent exposure to the bee pollen may energize them. They can run faster, etc. They may never suspect, sometime later when they become ill, that the same substance (now causing a stage 2 or 3 reaction) leads to fatigue or worse. Fifteen years ago, when I tried bee pollen, it swelled my throat immediately. Some nutritionists continually tout new foods that will energize, alleviate arthritis, etc. Sometimes they may have nutrients not readily available; often, it is a new food, not eaten before by most people. However, the small, alarm reaction that initially occurs can momentarily energize or alleviate arthritis via the adrenal output of a small stage 1 reaction. As stage 2 or 3 may soon arise, these panaceas are short-lived (and there is a new one every year). Rotating new foods can prevent stage 2 or 3 from occurring, of course. But if a food causes euphoria or increased energy, be careful.

One can be in different stages for different allergies. The general stress theory vis-a-vis allergy may give us insight into drug use too. As drugs are foreign to the body and toxic, an alarm reaction may occur to any drug when first used. It may alleviate symptoms again by an adrenal rush! But soon for reasons of toxicity or allergy, stage 2 or 3 will be reached. The allergic individual soon reacts negatively to virtually *all* drugs. One last word on the stress concept. It may be difficult to distinguish general stress from specific stressors. Selye lists migraines as due to general stress. This is incorrect. Those who abide by an allergy- and Candida-elimination diet soon become migraine-free regardless of their stress load! In health and science, many fail to separate the general from the specific, the theoretical from the experimental or clinical. My background as a physicist is always helpful to me in this regard.

Remember that chemical and pollen allergy have the same masking and withdrawal aspects as food allergy. Painters are known to travel many miles to get a whiff, if they're on vacation. When someone says "other people's perfume affects me, but mine is O.K.," they are masked for their own perfume which must also be eliminated. Be careful if testing your own allergies, experientially. A masked food, when avoided for 5 days, can show a full alarm reaction if tested at that time! This author had to be rushed to the hospital, when he tested himself (in this manner) for tomatoes. If only MBT had been known, instead!

Our international lecture tours have led to many fascinating "chemical adventures." Did you know that several nations reserve the right to spray pesticide on you before you land in their country? We found this out in Australia and New Zealand. The crew's actions on these flights also led to a few incidents. On the two flights with Australia's well-known international carrier, several crew members continued to smoke in areas forbidden to them (and near me) and also while preparing the food. These acts are against regulations. We got nowhere with them. The author then got metaphorical. As I was "pissed off," I (a lowly economy passenger) announced that I was going to relieve myself in the first class bathroom. The male attendants then chased after me and pounded on the door. They proclaimed that I was committing a great offense, far exceeding their poisoning me? On my next flight with the leading New

Zealand carrier, one crew member took his life in his hands by smoking in designated non-smoking areas (near me). We will attempt to fly on other carriers henceforth!

5

THE FIRST WEIGHT LOSS SCIENCE

Let's examine how allergy and related topics can cause weight gain *REGARDLESS OF CALORIC INTAKE.* This represents for the first time, all the non-caloric causes of weight gain ever to be spelled out in one place. First we'll list these factors, then explain them. Finally, you can see some results from our "before and after photos".

CAUSES OF WEIGHT GAIN AND/OR ADDICTION

1. Hypoglycemia. This can lead to a craving of sweets or any (allergic) substance that affects blood sugar. If you eat a meal and *then* have to have sweets, some food has dropped your blood sugar; presumably by an allergic response affecting your pancreas.

2. Candidiasis. See the next chapter for more details. Here cravings may be foods that contain simple carbohydrates and/or molds.

3. Faulty appestat. The turn on/turn off cells in the Appetite Control Center (appestat) in the hypothalamus in the brain may be malfunctioning from histamine or other allergic mediators. *Instead of turning off, they turn on as the allergic food is eaten.* So one gets *hungrier,* not satiated as one eats an offending food. Some people can't stop until they run out of the final frontier — space.

4. Disordered methionine metabolism.[10] This essential amino acid is improperly metabolized in many people. *Toxic, addictive, endorphin-like* substances may be produced. This may explain why many people eat only a few foods. They experience some kind of "high" from these foods. This is from the endorphin (opium-like) effects on the brain. Foods that don't elicit this reaction aren't eaten. But the resulting endorphin-like substances are toxic to the brain, liver, pancreas, etc. A vicious cycle begins.

5. Exorphins. Certain foods have recently been found to contain exorphins — opium-like substances *already formed in the food*. This mechanism doesn't depend on a disordered metabolism as the last mechanism did. Wheat gluten, milk casein and legumes (such as peanuts) are exorphin proteins. Giving up wheat and dairy are often crucial to losing weight. How many people do you know that don't crave these two or the ultimate, addictive food — pizza?

6. Disordered water metabolism. This mechanism may not involve addiction, only allergy. Here allergic mediators may affect the hypothalamus-pituitary-kidney-heart link that regulates water metabolism and blood pressure. Does your urine vary in density and color? Do you get thirsty after eating certain (non-salty) foods? Assuming no involvement of drugs, vitamins, salt, etc., this is likely due to allergic reactions. Eating allergic foods may cause you to retain water and the urine is darker and less urination occurs. Avoiding these foods resets the water regulation and diuresis (large urinary loss) results with a clear urine demonstrated. The large weight loss, early in a fast, is probably due to this resetting. When the author's allergies were bad a single tomato could lead to a water retention of several gallons. Avoiding this food then led to a large water (and weight) loss. The author once lost 6 pounds in an hour!

7. Carbohydrate craving due to low serotonin. Low serotonin (a neurotransmitter) is associated with depression. For the body to make serotonin from the amino acid, tryptophan, car-

bohydrates are needed. Excess protein and insufficient carbohydrates (a Candida diet, according to some experts) can lead to low serotonin levels. A carbohydrate binge may result as the body attempts to alleviate the depression associated with low serotonin.

8. Cell membrane fluidity. The cell membrane's fatty constituents lose their structural integrity during addictive and withdrawal phases. Nerve and blood cells are said to be readily affected. This too then is part of the cellular basis of addictive stress.

9. Viruses. Swiss researchers believe they have identified chronic, low-level viral titres that are linked to weight gain. Some of these researchers even believe that these viruses are transmittable. Chronic viruses also cause chemical and electromagnetic allergies. Special "zapper" electrical devices, available from the author, are effective in eliminating viruses.

10. Clogged gall bladder or bile duct. A liver/gall bladder flush can be performed here to help unclog this organ or the duct. Contact us for this information.

Now, all those who can't lose weight by watching calories can be comforted; and with the knowledge from this chapter, they should finally have success. Some weight loss centers have admitted to us that they sometimes work simply because they charge so much! The client is desperate to get his money's worth. But their failures are legion. With our methods, success often occurs *without* having to eat small amounts of food! It might shock those who have fought the weight battle for years, but *if non-allergenic foods are eaten, one feels satiated after very small amounts*. But, that slight "high" from endorphins or exorphins will be missing and may take some getting used to. (See the back of the book for our self-hypnosis/relaxation tape about quick help for overcoming addictions and staying on your diet.)

We should note that these mechanisms can in some cases cause underweight conditions and can occur from chemical and even pollen allergy, etc. Allergy testing and avoidance to counteract these mechanisms is crucial.

In more detail, the first thing the unsuccessful dieter needs is complete testing for allergies, Candidiasis and related factors. Food allergies that cause water retention or bingeing must be avoided. Avoid simple carbohydrates, do eat the complex carbohydrates—they're best anyway. This will help avoid hypoglycemic and Candida problems. Most people need to avoid dairy, peanut products and wheat as they contain the addictive exorphins. Many others find tomatoes and beef need to be avoided. Watch for changes in the color and amount of your urine to help determine which foods affect your water metabolism. Then you shouldn't need us to tell you what to do about those foods. After an initial avoidance, most foods can be eaten again. Just watch for the frequency. If you start to crave them everyday, you should also know what that means. That's right! And *you're* starting to become the expert on Allergies and Candida—as it should be!

Keep a diary, if you're not sure of what food and psychological factors may cause bingeing or water retention. Learn to be honest with yourself. Anything you crave or eat everyday may be the cause of your weight problems. Do get all the help and support that you need to help you stick to these—the *first scientific*— weight loss guidelines!

Pictured on the next page are some before and after photos given to us by two clients. The before photos are not full-body because some people are too shy (because of their weight) to take such photos. An interesting thing is that these ladies look years younger in the "after" photos than they did in the "before" photos, when they actually *were* years younger! These women lost all excess weight without any calorie counting at all. Muscle testing (you'll be able to do this soon) found all their "hidden" allergies. They then avoided these foods. They found it easy to love the foods that were good for them and to give up their former addictions. They look better because these hidden allergies were also affecting their health, even if it was "subclinical."

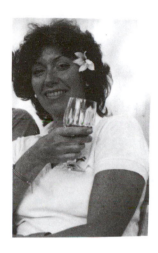

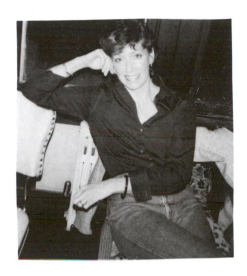

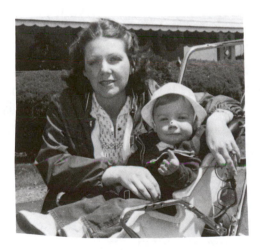

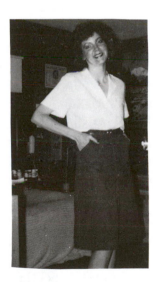

Figures 4-7.
HEBS "FIRST SCIENCE OF WEIGHT LOSS" results. The "before" pictures are on the left and the "after" photos are on the right.

6

ALLERGY TO CHEMICALS, VITAMINS, GERMS, & ENERGIES

Complete allergy testing should include foods, inhalants, chemicals and energy allergy. *INHALANTS*, include dust, mold, grass, tree and weed pollens, insects and animal epithelia. It helps to know which pollens are "in season" in your area as these can cause any symptom. Orthodox physicians say they are stymied in finding out why Rheumatoid Arthritis strikes many children in the Spring and Summer (when tree and grass pollens are in the air). Maybe one day, they'll read the literature from the allergists! Any allergy can cause any symptom! If winter is a problem, indoor dust and mold may be the culprit. Dust on heating elements (radiators) becomes the even more allergenic, fried dust.

One class of chemicals, *PHENOLS*, deserves special attention. These ubiquitous chemicals include artificial colors, flavors and preservatives, the greenish lining in canned foods, and medical preservatives such as in allergy or vitamin injections. Some physicians have claimed that allergy injections have never been proven to be safe and effective.[11] (Allergy symptoms typically change as children grow up; shots may be irrelevant at best.) Most fruits and some nuts also contain salicylates (made famous by the Feingold diet for hyperactive children), which are a subset of phenol compounds. Our own hormones and neurotransmitters are made up from amino acids which are often phenol compounds too. Compounds called indoles and scatoles made by intestinal bacteria are also phenol compounds.

This can lead to special problems. There are two possibilities. First, one can become *allergic to one's own hormones or neurotransmitters*. Secondly, the body may *run out of enzymes* to break down these substances, due to overload of phenols. The body continuously builds up (anabolizes) substances and breaks them down (catabolism). These are the two components of metabolism. But if the body becomes allergic to, or is unable to catabolize, its hormones and neurotransmitters, any hormonal or neurological symptom can result. Many cases of PMS (Premenstrual Syndrome) may involve phenol allergy or metabolic overload as progesterone is a phenol compound. Other such compounds, in the body, include epinephrine (adrenalin), norepinephrine (noradrenalin), dopamine, acetylcholine, serotonin, and uric acid. When unusual amounts of hormones or neurotransmitters are present in the body, various endocrine, neurological or emotional symptoms may result. Minimizing external phenol compounds and some treatment or balancing for phenol allergy or overload is needed.

A frequently overlooked allergy is *NUTRITIONAL SUPPLEMENT ALLERGY*. People spend small fortunes in the hope of getting well. Nutritional "experts" often ignore this problem. Too many in holistic health view supplements, herbs, etc. the same way orthodox physicians view drugs. Potential side effects don't enter their minds. As more people experience the ineffectiveness of conventional medicine, they may encounter the hazards of "natural" therapy. Each of us must take the responsibility of learning as much as we can about what is happening to us. And MBT shines as the quickest way to ascertain allergies to everything including supplements.

We need to know three things about potential allergy to

supplements. One is the nature of the nutrient. E.g.. the amino acid tryptophan is a phenolic compound. Two, what it is derived from. And three, the excipients (non-nutritional ingredients) that are in the tablet or capsule. Excipients include fillers, binders, coatings, lubricants, preservatives, etc. Until the last 10 years all Vitamin (**Vit.**) C was synthesized from glucose molecules derived from corn. The prevalence of corn allergy led to the present availability of Vitamin C derived from sago palm and tapioca. The latter, the sole item in its food family, may be best tolerated. (Sago palm is in the date family.) And Vit. C allergy *can* lead to bladder and kidney problems. We side here some- what with orthodox physicians, though they don't understand the problem completely. Except for tapioca Vit. C., all Vit. C led to bladder and kidney problems in this author. Frequent, burning urination and even stones resulted. I found the cause; it was a uric acid problem. Physicians can check for *low* blood levels of uric acid. Uric acid is filtered out by the kidneys at one point. If it is not reabsorbed, (despite imbibing much water) the passing of these crystals in the urine results in the above excruciating symptoms. Hidden parasitosis is often the ultimate cause of bladder problems.

Let's look at vitamin sources. Natural Vitamin E is derived from wheat (usually) or soy or synthetic sources (petrochemi- cals). As unnatural as it sounds, the last may be the best tolerated. It may go through more purification stages than the naturally derived E. Vits. A and D may come from fish. Beta-carotene (pro-Vitamin A) may come from carrots or synthetic sources. Lecithin comes from soy, eggs or beef. Inositol comes from corn and choline bitartrate is derived from grapes. Bran can come from wheat (usually) or oats, rice and corn. Some digestive enzymes and other supplements come from the fungus, Asper- gillus. Betaine hydrochloride comes from beets. Let's look at minerals next. Gluconates & fumarates come from corn. Amino acid chelates come from soy. Lactates/orotates come from milk. Bioflavonoids are usually derived from citrus sources (probably lemon). An algae based source — quercitin — is available. The B-Vitamins, biotin, folic acid and B12 are derived from fermentation of bacteria. *BACTERIAL ALLERGY* is cited in the older allergy texts. It can cause asthma, GI and neurological or emotional symptoms. Some cheeses, like Swiss, have bacterial as well as mold cultures. If a multivitamin or yeast-free B-Complex repeats (or comes up) it is probably due to bacterial allergy. Acidophilus supplements are, of course, bacteria too. Citric acid and calcium ascorbate may be yeast fermented. Intestinal cleansers may be a problem. Bentonite is basically earth and will have molds. Psyllium is a grass.

Natural food glaze may (or may not be listed) as a coating on tablets. This can come from corn, crude petroleum or the lac resin. The lac is a bug which lives on trees. Anyone with tree, insect or dust allergy may react to this. Dust allergy is really allergy to the mites which grow on dead and flaked-off skin. Alfalfa is a grass to which many are allergic. Amino acids may come from milk, yeast, beef or vegetable sources. Capsules are derived from beef or pork (gelatin) and may contain preservatives. Taking a supplement everyday predisposes to allergy. But supplements can be rotated too.

Let's look more deeply into *CHEMICAL ALLERGY*. In today's world, many are reacting to their clothing, furniture, beds, carpets, walls, toiletries, perfumes, cigarette smoke, cleaners, reading materials, pesticides,[12] etc. Homes and work places have become toxic. Studies have shown that housewives are more cancer prone than women who work elsewhere. The indoor pollution from the above items is the likely culprit.[13] Other studies show that indoor pollution in our homes and work places is worse than outdoor pollution, even in dirty cities. We have been brainwashed into cleaning our rugs, floors, sinks, ovens, toilets, cars, homes and even ourselves with toxic, allergic substances. Who bothers to read the small print that says, "use only in well ventilated areas?" And is there a well ventilated area? In the U.S., especially since the Arab oil embargo of 1973, we've rushed into over-insulating our homes. A house used to change or recycle its air every half hour. Now the air is unchanged for three or more hours. Some insulation materials, like formaldehyde, led to their own nightmares. We've also been brainwashed into smelling like (artificial) flowers. Per-fumes, colognes, underarm deodorants, shampoos, soaps, hair sprays, douches, room fresheners, toilet paper — anything that comes in contact with us — must smell "right." Even mail is sent out perfumed. In some holistic circles, people feel they must burn perfumed incense before meetings. HEBS consultants routinely see people taking the most powerful, toxic (and inef-fective) drugs for headaches. MBT often indicates all that is needed is to stop using scented products! Many are unaware of the effects of their own perfume due to the masking effect.

Rugs are great offenders to the human ecology; often contain-ing hundreds of toxic chemicals. These include pesticides and fungicides (and formaldehyde) that take months or years to outgas. West Germany may lead the world in the study of the "Sick Building Syndrome." This misnomer (it's the people that get sick) refers to the allergic, toxic effects of newer building and insulating materials on people.

Other chemical sources include pesticides (at home or in food), on-the-job chemicals, drugs, anesthetics, and food addi-tives. Pesticides are usually neurotoxins. But a human nerve cell is very similar to an insect nerve cell! That our nerve cells are infinitely more intricately connected only serves to point out their increased fragility and vulnerability. Canned food contains lead and phenol. Paints and gasoline may contain lead. Our livestock is force-fed antibiotics, hormones and tranquilizers that will enter our bodies too. American meat is banned in some European countries. Fish is often treated with antibiotics and formaldehyde by the fishermen and the supermarkets. Fresh produce is waxed and treated with other chemicals. Ammonia and other toxic cleaners are allowed to come in contact with the food we eat. Sadly, for every chemical used there is either no need or a more natural alternative.

Our water supplies are a major health hazard. Industrial seepage, human sewage, chlorine, fluorine and other chemicals are found in most tap water. Fluorine is already present in natural and sufficient amounts in water. The extra 1 PPM (part per million) is a great health threat. Some nations, e.g. India and Italy, *remove* fluorine from their tap water. Most European countries have banned water fluoridation while phony studies by the industrial-pharmaceutical-medical-dental complex attempt to dupe the American people. This is the usual, orthodox, medical method of counteracting the effects of one poison (here, sugar) with another poison.

Chlorine, in our polluted water, combines with other chemicals to make trihalomethanes, including chloroform. The latter is depicted in the movies when a treated handkerchief is used to render a foe unconscious. A recent major N.Y. newspaper article warned readers not to take lengthy, hot showers because of all the chloroform emitted.[14]

Pharmaceutical, recreational and illicit drug use is rampant in our society. We consider alcohol, nicotine and marijuana to be drugs. Cocaine use is now epidemic in the U.S. People take these substances to "alter their moods." But it is probably some combination of hypoglycemia, allergies and Candidiasis (**HAC**) that has already altered their moods (negatively) causing them to seek an even more dangerous remedy. Further poisoning oneself is not the answer. Over-the-counter and prescription medicines are standardly used to mask symptoms while the cause of the malady is ignored. This is not Science! Nutritional supplements and energy balancing could obviate the need for taking most pharmaceuticals. Balancing the ecology could even obviate the need for some supplements.

Now, let's explore the new realm of *ENERGY ALLERGY;* often unknown, or unrecognized by, many ecologists. This is another area where kinesiologists lead the way. You can indeed be sensitive to, and harmed by, colors, fluorescents, T.V.'s, computer terminals, household A.C. currents and overhead lines, microwaves (ovens and antennae), electric watches, LED's or LCD's (Light Emitting Diodes and Liquid Crystal Displays) other electromagnetic radiation, sounds, etc. Perhaps only with muscle testing can one so quickly determine energy allergy. Blood sugars may even be affected by energy allergy! This author has found that chronic viruses—secondary to parasitosis—cause *electromagnetic allergies.* Such sensitivity or toxicity is now commonplace, even if unsuspected. People who work near microwave antennae or at computer terminals have a very high rate of cataract formation at young ages. Just from wearing an LCD watch, I had marked pain in my hamstrings for two years! Fortunately, a kinesiologist tested for this and the problem was soon corrected. You will never know unless you can test all the possibilities. Many people can't safely wear certain colors or gold or silver or electric watches. There may never be a skin reaction, but imbalance and illness will result.This author feels best when wearing a certain shade of green or plain white. Many with ecological illness seem to appear wearing purple. This could be allergy/addiction! Soon you will know how to test *all* environmental factors.

Fluorescent lighting has become ubiquitous in the work place. Many people "space out" or poorly perform tasks under them. Such lighting is *discontinuous* and unnatural. The brain is adversely affected by such a flickering light source. We need to be surrounded by *continuous, full spectrum light.* Fluorescents lack parts of the light spectrum especially in the violet and ultraviolet ranges. The latter was meant to actually enter through the eye and even the skull and positively affect the pineal gland. This gland directs the hypothalamus which directs the pituitary and hence the endocrine system. The endocrine, neurological and immune systems all interact. So mood, sleep and energy can all be affected by lack of ultraviolet light.[15] Research is under way to prove this. The recent term S.A.D. (Seasonal Affected Disorder) refers to the syndrome of depression and fatigue that plagues many workers during winter months when they receive a deficiency of sunlight. The ultraviolet also helps the body to make Vit. D which is needed for proper calcium metabolism. Now several companies offer "full spectrum fluorescent lights." These are a big improvement, but probably fail to correct another problem. Fluorescent fixtures emit very intense sound waves that are in an inaudible frequency range. It is said to be as intense as a jet flying 100 feet overhead. Sometimes you may hear fluorescents "bleed" into the audible range. As with the light from the fluorescents, what you don't consciously hear may well adversely affect you.

Eyeglasses, sunglasses and contact lens will also screen out the needed full spectrum of light. Tinted lenses invariably weaken people. Even our windows screen out full spectrum light. My old public school had windows that clearly had flowed downwards. (Glass is a "semi-liquid.") New, "improved" glass doesn't flow, but it doesn't allow for the full spectrum either.

Room or clothing colors can also adversely affect you. These also act as filters allowing primarily the color you see to enter the body. Clinical studies have proven that pink weakens and blue may energize. Pink is now used in prisons and mental institutions. Weightlifters try to be in blue rooms. Each color has a different effect on each organ as each organ has a different optimum frequency. This is also true of the acupuncture meridians and even the different spinal vertebrae.

Color T.V.'s and black-and-whites can cause imbalance. A color T.V. is always "on" as long as it's plugged in! (Again, intense inaudible sound waves are said to be emitted.) T.V.'s also emit flickering light, more readily seen in a movie showing a T.V. While some epileptics can get convulsions from such flickering light, many others experience "subclinical" effects including spaceyness, fatigue and sleep problems. (Of course with T.V., it could be the program.) Any prolonged stress can weaken the immune system. Medical testing is geared only to ascertaining the occurrence of long term, exposure-induced, medical illness; not the immediate, subclinical effects we've discussed.

Microwave ovens will leak "a little bit" and they also alter the food, creating free radicals. (See Ch. 13.) Many, with E.I. test weak to microwaved food. Virtually all books on Candida ignore this fact — they don't have MBT! A miniscule leak may well cause energy imbalance (as indicated by MBT). We will examine energy imbalance in later chapters; for now, let's say that such imbalance is a definite stress to the whole body.

Household A.C. current and overhead high tension wires create "unnatural" magnetic fields. The conservative New Englanders were the last to allow overhead wires in their community because they felt "funny" under them. There may even be electromagnetic pollution that you haven't heard about. Both Eastern and Western military researchers are investigating the use of Extremely Low Frequency (ELF) electromagnetic waves, ostensibly for submarine communication. These waves can go through the earth. Physicist colleagues have told me that the Soviets and Americans may be beaming these waves to each other's cities?!

The Chernobyl explosion has enabled the world to see the dangers of radioactivity. European HEBS graduates have told this author that many people are reporting "subclinical" ills (verifiable via MBT) even though their governments said the dose was "too low to affect them." But short term energy imbalance can lead to long term medical illness. There are radioactive sources in our everyday lives that need to be identified. Some smoke detectors emit radiation. Older watches used a radioactive substance to fluoresce in the dark. Workers who used their tongues to wet the brushes that placed these substances on the dials had a high cancer mortality rate. Medical and dental X-rays have a history of higher dosages and abuse.

Many areas of the U.S. contain soil with a naturally high content of radioactive radon gas. Air currents can bring it, and trap it, in homes. The FDA has approved the use of irradiation of food despite the fact that it destroys enzymes and nutrients, creates toxins, and alters the food irrevocably. Even dangerous mutations of germs, including Candida, could conceivably occur. Our purpose throughout this chapter is not to frighten the reader; rather to make you aware so you can test and also make the appropriate personal and political choices. We, the cells and molecules we are made of, were meant to be in electromagnetic harmony with our surroundings. What you can't see can harm you.

We also need to be in harmony with the *sounds* around us. Sounds from fluorescents, T.V.'s, refrigerators, furnaces, air conditioners, computers, air filters, etc, can cause "sound allergy" if you will. Planes, trains, highway, home appliances and nearby industrial noises can affect us. Some, like T.V.'s and fluorescents and some bug killer devices emit intense but inaudible sound waves. But these can nonetheless throw you off kilter. Now all of our cells emit and receive electromagnetic radiation (light waves or photons). But our cells also emit and receive sound waves or phonons. And a harmony must be maintained here too. Physicists are moving into the field of energy medicine. Fancy machines that test and balance with lasers, monochromatic light, electricity and sound are being utilized. But muscle testing and balancing is available to everyone now.

The music we listen to can have profound effects on us. The rock beat (soft-soft-*hard*) is very weakening to virtually everyone! But the waltz beat (*hard*-soft-soft or 1-2-3) is very strengthening. Popular music since the 50's became more unnatural every year. And it all fits in — the warped music is apparently very addictive to the young! The ubiquitous headphones are worn in school, on the street and while doing (or attempting) homework. This author believes that the concept of allergy-addiction extends *beyond* foods and chemicals. It pertains to chemicals, energies, T.V.'s, rock music. We've seen pets included too. John Diamond, M.D., has found that digitally recorded (discontinuous) music is weakening. Digitally recorded tapes, records and CD's are now commonplace. Different organs are again preferentially affected by different frequencies as detectable by MBT and other tests.

We are also in harmony with the *electrical charges* around us. We need the proper balance of positive to negative *IONS* in our vicinity. An ion is just a charged atom or molecule in the air — one that has lost its neutrality by gaining or losing electrons (which are negatively charged.) The natural ratio of ions is 3 to 2, positive to negative. Forced air systems (which also can contain much dust and mold), weather fronts,[16] air conditioners, even cooking can place excess positive ions in the air around you. Obtaining a negative ion generator may be helpful.

Synthetic clothing will trap these harmful excess positive ions around you. Synthetic clothing has been proven to affect blood pressure.[17] Many people feel irritable wearing synthetics. Use only cotton, silk or linen for all clothing, bedding, etc. Try to get untreated cotton, i.e., cotton not permanent pressed, sanforized or otherwise treated. These are often pressed on with formaldehyde. You can test for untreated cotton with a water dropper. A drop of water will be quickly absorbed by untreated cotton; but it will bead up for a while if chemicals are present.

Let's return to heating systems. Gas should be avoided according to the father of clinical ecology, Theron Randolph, M.D. Gas lines and stoves all leak enough to bother those with E.I. Randolph recommends turning the gas off outside the house. Kerosene and gasoline heaters obviously emit toxic chemicals. Low temperature portable radiators are sold to prevent dust-frying. Wood stoves can bother anyone with tree or fungus allergy. Fungus grows on most trees. Some people are even bothered by their (unheated) Christmas trees.

Given this information, calmly decide what factors in your environment you can change and how you'll live with the others. You see why it's wise to change what you can (diet?) right away.

7

CANDIDA ALBICANS AND ITS HUMAN INTERACTION

W e come now to the complicated, and not well-understood topic of the role of Candida albicans in chronic illness. Environmental physicians believe that overgrowth of Candida albicans may be a cause of much chronic, degenerative, immunological and "emotional" illness. This includes allergy itself. But this chapter will also introduce the revolutionary concept that energy imbalance induced by Candida can also cause these ills—in many cases without much overgrowth! Regarding allergies, recall that many allergies arise for other reasons including too frequent exposure (including ingestion) of the allergens. And chemical sensitivities we shall see in the next chapter can be due to the Epstein-Barr Virus. So a key to the role of Candida albicans (**C.a.**) will be universal food allergies and/or multiple pollen allergies.

We should note that Candida albicans and other fungus and other germs are found in everyone's colon. It's also found in the air and on food. A day after birth nearly all infants have a positive skin reaction indicating exposure to Candida albicans. Thus only when overgrowth (or energy imbalance) occurs does illness ensue.

Let's start by listing possible symptoms of Candidiasis. Again allergies, other infectious agents and other factors may cause any of these symptoms. Again, the reader is advised that *Protozoan parasites are often the underlying key factor. Parasites can weaken the person leading to Candidiasis or exist instead of Candida.*

POSSIBLE SYMPTOMS OF CANDIDIASIS[18]
Female disorders, including vaginitis, PMS, endometriosis   (the

bacterium-like germ, chlamydia, may be at fault here), ovarian or uterine fibroids, sterility, infertility

Male disorders, including prostatitis

Allergies

G.I.: Coated tongue, bad breath, gas, bloating, pain, diarrhea, colitis, ileitis, constipation, ulcers, diaper rash, thrush

Fungal nails, athlete's foot (other fungi are usually causative here)

Skin conditions, acne, psoriasis

Heart: Arrhythmias, Mitral Valve Prolapse, Low or High Blood Pressure, the author's discovery of "dyslexic heart"

Dyslexia (another HEBS discovery), hyperactivity

Neurological and Neuromuscular: headaches, migraines, fatigue, spaceyness, poor memory (often for names), poor balance, amnesia, M.S. (Multiple Sclerosis)

Addictions, especially sweets and yeast-containing foods

Emotional, e.g. schizophrenia

Earaches, especially in young children

Asthma, sinusitis (If nutrition and diet change don't help with these two, C.a. may be involved)

Bladder and kidney problems

Immune deficiency

Autoimmune disease, e.g. lupus

Endocrine disorders, e.g., thyroid problems (Cryptocides – see the next chapter – may be at fault here)

Problem pregnancy

Problems with any moist, mucous membrane

Vitreous floaters in the eyes (This fluid in the eye gelling up and casting shadows against the retina.) This is known to occur in people with high blood sugar

Low or high blood sugar

Structural imbalance in the spine, cranium or jaw

Candida septicemia – the medical term for C.a. in the blood

We're ready to examine the reasons for the present epidemic

of Candidiasis.

POSSIBLE CAUSES OF CANDIDIASIS

1. Antibiotics
2. Birth Control Pills
3. Cortisone drugs
4. Excess sweets — sucrose is the worst
5. Excess yeast containing foods, nutrient-poor food
6. Artificial or junk food
7. Starvation (Candidiasis is also rampant in starving Africa)
8. Foods with heated oils or other free radicals
9. Allergies. While C.a. can cause allergies, the reverse can be true too as toxins released from chronic allergies can weaken the immune system
10. Sexual or intimate contact can pass this germ
11. Other infectious agents, including the ones discussed in the next chapter
12. Endocrine disorders
13. Toxicities
14. Radiation
15. Any immune system stress
16. Fluoride toxicity
17. Genetic Predisposition
18. Pregnancy
19. Environmental mold exposure, either in your home (basement or bathroom) or local geographical area such as in humid areas
20. Excess nutritional supplementation. These may feed the yeast as they have similar nutritional needs, including some B-vitamins, iron, zinc
21. Old age
22. Emotional stress
23. Immune deficiency, e.g., low levels of (s)IgA
24. Fetal immune system tricked while forming by presence of mother's overgrowth.

Let's expand upon some of the causes of the epidemic of Candidiasis. We have used an excellent series of tapes from the 1985 Yeast-Human Interaction Conference as a main source here.[19] Medical experts believe that over ⅔ of the population of the U.S. suffers from chronic Candidiasis. The leading culprit is thought to be *ANTIBIOTICS*. Sometimes, just one episode of taking antibiotics (or the birth control pill) initiates a lifetime of unfolding misery! This could be prevented if the measures below were taken.

Antibiotics will kill bacteria that may (or may not) be harming you; but they will also kill the friendly flora that live in our intestines. These helpful bacteria, such as the acidophilus strains, compete with any intestinal fungus and other germs and thus keep them from overgrowing. The acidophilus perform many other useful functions such as making vitamins and enzymes and their own antibiotics. But most antibiotic medications will kill off the acidophilus allowing the yeast a major victory.

Now antibiotics have saved countless lives in the last 50 years or so, but today they are terribly abused by Western physicians. Often a cold is really a viral infection (or even misdiagnosed allergies) and anti-bacterial medication is totally inappropriate. The proper procedure of taking a culture is rarely done. Antibiotics are also found in great amounts in American meats and have even led to the mutating of new strains of antibiotic-resistant bacteria! Routinely handing out antibiotics has become an international tragedy of tragic proportions and has led to perhaps the major iatrogenic (doctor-caused) illness on the planet — Candidiasis. Our immune system at its best has a tough time against fungus. The extra help it gets from the friendly flora should not be obviated. Certainly physicians should prescribe acidophilus during or after antibiotic use — but most don't. This imbalance in the human ecology can initiate an unfolding of much chronic suffering in the human host.

The birth control pill is composed of progesterone-like hormones that, as a side effect, alter the vaginal mucosa allowing Candida to overgrow. Yeast favor dark, moist or humid places whether it's in or on the body or in your basement. Increased progesterone is also released during pregnancy, accounting for the frequent vaginal infections many women experience at that time.

Cortisone drugs weaken the immune system — they're used for this purpose in organ transplants — and also raise the blood sugar. Yeast also have receptors for similar type substances, so for all these reasons, this type of medication also favors yeast overgrowth. Mercury dental fillings[20]— the so-called "silver amalgam" — have been found to be neurotoxic, immunotoxic and even antibiotic. The Swedish Dental Academy, in 1986, admitted it had made a terrible mistake and harmed the population. Studies, by Swedish metallurgists, had proved that about half of the mercury leaches out of the fillings within a few years!! They began banning the use of mercury in fillings. (This was done by the American Dental Society in the 1840's before corruption arose.) Bacteria and fungus in the mouth can convert mercury into methylmercury which is even more toxic and antibiotic. The last fact means your acidophilus can again be killed. Many with Environmental Illness have had their amalgams replaced. Substitutes include porcelain-ceramic type material, plastics, and gold. The ceramics include P-10, P-30, Herculite, and Occlusin. There may be no perfect solution. Most ceramics also contain some metal. Visio-fil is a plastic supposedly without any metals. Gold is a metal and can cause energy imbalance in the head (and allergy). We recommend against any and all metals. One thing you can do is to use muscle testing with a sample before replacements are done. We also recommend against root canals and crowns as these can cause the gums or teeth to become infected.

There is much in modern diets that can lead to yeast overgrowth. The average diet is said to contain 100 times the sugar content that our grandparents ate at the turn of the century. Sucrose is the worst form of sugar and the favorite of the yeast. Sucrose is different from all other sugars and is called invert sugar. Yeast have much of the enzyme, invertase, which metabolizes sucrose. So eating foods with sucrose is feeding Candida's "sweet tooth." Any concentrated sweet can feed a yeast overgrowth. Fruits are replete with simple sugars. Melons are said to be one of the worst. They may have much mold content. Honey, maple syrup, rice syrup, etc. are other sweeteners to avoid. Other sugars include anything that ends in -ose (like glucose), or -ol (like sorbitol). Although the -ol's will be more complex than the -ose's. Clinical ecologists had recommended a diet of less than 60 grams a day of carbohydrate. These carbohydrates would be complex — like grains and potatoes — and not simple carbohydrates — like fruits or sugar. And some would even resort to a carbohydrate-free diet if this failed. These severe carbohydrate restrictions are now losing favor. But if Candidiasis exists, only complex carbohydrates (if any) would be allowed.

Today's diet is also high in foods containing yeast and mold. You will need to avoid these foods to overcome a Candida problem or mold allergy.

FOODS CONTAINING YEAST AND MOLDS
1.Cheese and other milk products
2. Alcoholic beverages
3. Anything aged, fermented, or malted
4. Vinegar or anything containing vinegar (mustard, ketchup, mayonnaise, salad dressings, pickles)
5. Soy sauce, tamari
6. Dried fruits
7. Mushrooms
8. MSG (Monosodium Glutamate)
9. Tofu and sprouts (sit in water)
10. Baker's yeast (in baked goods) Bacterial cultures and baking soda can be used as a substitute, to make dough rise
11. Brewer's yeast. Brewer's yeast may be found in vitamin supplements (and alcoholic beverages) and was a major factor that nearly led to the author's untimely demise.
12. Foods that pick up molds during their processing and storing

These can include peanuts and other nuts, grains, herbs, spices. (Peanuts also contain the potent carcinogen aflatoxin — a mold product.)

13. Anything that exposes much surface area can attract mold and other germs. This is why hamburger meat may cause a problem while steak may not

14. Similarly, any food left in the open for too long can pick up molds, etc.

We list below the four classes of foods to avoid if chronic Candidiasis exists.

FOUR CLASSES OF FOODS TO AVOID

1. Sweets.
2. Foods containing yeast or mold.
3. Any allergic food.
4. Foods containing heated oils and other free radicals.

This may be the only reference to warn readers of the dangers of the fourth class of foods above. This class of foods includes fried food and also any food containing free radicals. See Ch. 13. Some people need to eliminate or reduce even unheated oils and fats. We've actually seen women who've had a return of vaginal Candidiasis after eating one potato chip! And they weren't allergic to the potatoes. (Do you crave fried food?) Again we are the first to include microwaved food, as a class of foods to avoid, due to the free radicals it contains — see Ch. 13. Most Candidiasis sufferers *will* have to abide by these diet restrictions, for some time, if they want to get well. However, the length of time for severe diet restrictions — an individual matter — can be dramatically shortened by the energy balancing methods in this book. Our revolutionary discoveries also reveal that many E.I. sufferers may not have much overgrowth. Rather they are suffering from (rapidly correctable) energy disturbances.

Nonetheless, you would be well advised to do your best to adhere to these anti-Candida diet guidelines. You may find yourself eating a lot of fish and vegetables. Don't overeat meats. You would stress your kidneys and digestive organs with excess protein and fats. Use Appendix C to find foods that are OK and that you want to eat. Find foods that will provide most of your calories from complex carbohydrates (starches). Remember, if you say there isn't anything there for you, it really means you have been used to getting high from foods that are really bad for you! Make some changes for the better now!

Breakfast appears to be a problem for some people. Again it's more conditioning. People feel guilty if they don't have cereal for breakfast. The reader should know that it was an American M.D. at the turn of the century who started this trend. His name was Kellogg—yes *that* Kellogg. The truth is your breakfast can be anything you would eat at any other time of the day. If you have the HAC syndrome, avoid the fruity breakfasts which have unfortunately been described in recent bestsellers. Always have some green vegetables with every meal, if possible. There should be some protein on your breakfast menu. No, we won't tell you precisely what to eat, because we haven't tested you for sensitivities. That's up to you with the kinesiological methods in a later chapter.

Let's return to our list of possible Candidiasis causors. Any prolonged or severe toxic exposure can weaken the immune system. This includes fluoride, radiation and artificial food. The recommendation of fluoridated water, toothpaste and vitamins is the usual American way of trying to compensate for one poison (here, sugar) with another poison. Fluoride, a necessary nutrient, is present in sufficient amounts in water and food. Excesses are very damaging to our cells.

The immune system is itself adversely affected by allergy mediators—the substances released from allergic reactions. Thus while Candidiasis can lead to universal allergies, continual allergic reactions can help lead to Candidiasis. Nutritional deficiencies lead to a weak immune system — Candidiasis is said to be rampant in starving African countries. But these countries also receive two American products in abundance — antibiotics and sugar. Fried, oily food and junk food weaken the immune system.

Sexual or intimate contact can spread the Candida organism from one partner to another. The male sex organ may harbor the yeast without any untoward signs but can reinfect the female organ. Enlightened gynecologists often treat the male partner of women with recurrent vaginal yeast infections. We have also seen that many women do not overcome this problem until all four classes of yeast-favoring foods are eliminated and the energy balancing is done.

Candida can cause endocrine disorders but the reverse is also true as the endocrine system is linked to the immune system. Many with Candidiasis have other chronic, undiagnosed infections including parasitic and viral disorders. (See the next chapter.) Sometimes, however, these other infections may occur first. Of course, a weak immune system is at the heart of all these infections including Candidiasis. Unchecked overgrowths of opportunistic organisms will ordinarily not occur if the human host has a good immune system. Supposedly we all have Herpes viruses, e.g., within us but most of us will not manifest with any symptoms.

There appears to be a definite genetic predisposition regarding this yeast disorder. Different genes are being found to control the body's ability to ward off different types of germs (bacteria, virus, fungus, etc.) Certain ethnic strains may have a weakness or predisposition towards Candidiasis. You may see evidence of several generations of it in some families.

ENVIRONMENTAL MOLD EXPOSURE is an insidious and potentially overwhelming stress. Recently, the University of Florida had a scandalous series of events with one of its new megastructures. Many of the faculty and students became so ill, they began wearing gas masks to their classes. After months of searching for many modern, toxic chemicals, mold toxins in the air system was found to be the culprit! Many people were left in a disabled condition. Presumably E.I. and Candidiasis resulted. The University had changed the air system at the last moment to save money. Molds love moist, dark places like air conditioning systems. It is interesting to note that anthropologists believe that man was "spawned" in the African desert — a mold free environment to be sure! It can be difficult to choose an agent to kill household mold. The agent may cause as much harm as the mold toxins. Don't use formaldehyde as one allergy book recommended. (We believe heart and brain function can be seriously affected by this chemical.) Try borax, Zephiran or chlorine; maybe you can get someone who doesn't have E.I. to do the job.

A novel idea is that *MEGADOSES OF NUTRIENTS MAY OCCASIONALLY PREFERENTIALLY FEED INTERNAL YEAST.* Most cells have some similar nutritional requirements. A vitamin for us may also be a vitamin for C.a. This includes some B-vitamins, iron, zinc and other nutrients. The "experts" often routinely prescribe these nutrients to supposedly help rid the body of Candida. Unfortunately, they do not have the tool — kinesiology — that you will soon have, to determine if a substance is beneficial or not!

As noted in the last chapter, the protective antibody (s)IgA is needed to coat the body's mucous membranes. A deficiency of this antibody could allow yeast or other opportunistic germs to flourish.

Some speculate that if C.a. crosses the placental barrier, it may incorporate itself into the fetus' primitive immune system and trick it into believing the yeast is part of the fetus. Antibodies to C.a. then would not be made. *ACETALDEHYDE* (similar to, and more toxic than, formaldehyde) from C.a. may also cross the placenta and lead to a weak immune system. In a later chapter, we hypothesize that yeast toxins from the mother can lead to hyperactivity and dyslexia in the fetus' later life. Many with Candidiasis may be the second or third generation with yeast-caused illness! Pregnant women must do all they can to avoid yeast infections and discharges. Vaginal discharges and subclinical yeast infections are so rampant that many gynecologists now tell their patients, "it's normal." This isn't true! Craving pickles and ice cream is not normal, and may be a hint of a yeast problem. Suffering through nine months of strict diet observance is less troublesome than years with a sickly or hyperactive child.

Lastly, Candida can be spread by household pets, especially cats. Veterinarians report Candidiasis in horses, dogs and cats. Sometimes antibiotics are again to blame. Even "healthy cats" apparently harbor C.a. and parasites (Toxoplasma). Physicians warn pregnant women not to change cat litter boxes. But maybe we should all take heed? Allergists have known that cat saliva is very allergenic and seems to last "forever." We have seen many with M.S. that began only after a cat was brought into the home. Cats even when healthy harbor much yeast and when they get leukemia, e.g. a significant overgrowth is often involved. Now let's look at some complaints due to Candida.

SYMPTOMS OF CANDIDIASIS

As the list indicates, any immunological, endocrine, neurological, metabolic or chronic, degenerative physical or emotional illness may result. A complete medical history and appropriate diagnostic tests can indicate if C.a. is the culprit. Chances are that if a patient's complaints are varied, complex and not in a pattern that the physician may have memorized in medical school, Candidiasis should be considered.

Medical dogma holds that Candidiasis is limited to oral thrush, vaginitis, fungal nails, athlete's foot, or Candida septicemia. The last is unchecked Candida growth in the blood which occurs in leukemia patients, and others, who have had their immune system further compromised with radiation or chemotherapy.

Now as fungus favor moist, mucous membranes; it is easy to see how C.a. can flourish anywhere in the G.I. tract — from the mouth (thrush) to the anus (diaper rash). The lungs (asthma) and sinuses can also become "hangouts." Clinical ecologists may recommend snorting or inhaling anti-fungal drugs to counteract yeast problems in these places. Mucous membranes under the skin and in the ear passage ways may also be favored by yeast if the local ecology or immune system are compromised.

Now C.a. can cause problems in the body *far* from where it may occur as an overgrowth. This is because its waste products may enter the blood and travel anywhere in the body. (Some earlier books on Candida mistakenly stated that actual, local yeast overgrowth was the only way for an organ to be affected.) Candida's toxins include carbon monoxide (as found by Stephen Levine, Ph.D.), alcohol, acetaldehyde, steroid substances and large molecules of unknown structure, simply called Candida toxins. Nearly 100 Candida-toxins are known.

In a seminal paper, in 1984, C. Orian Truss, M.D. — the father of the Candida hypothesis or at least the dissemination of this hypothesis — stated that acetaldehyde was the likely cause of most Candida associated illness.[21] This substance (pronounced acid-al-da-hide) is very toxic and volatile. Truss detailed how many metabolic, neurological, endocrine and "emotional" ills could result from acetaldehyde's effects on the body. Acetaldehyde also occurs in cigarettes, alcoholic beverages and smog (including auto exhaust). The liver has enzymes to detoxify this substance. These same enzymes would also detoxify formaldehyde — the smaller brother of acetaldehyde. Thus, the two together may overload the body's defenses. The E.I. are known to be very sensitive to formaldehyde. Later we shall see that this researcher has formulated an hypothesis which linked these two aldehydes as affecting "brain and heart integration." These have their own unfolding of illness.

This author believes that C.a. may be the cause of much hypoglycemia as follows. Low blood sugar may result from either a rapid growth of C.a. or paradoxically from the *"DIE-OFF EFFECT."* To examine this, we need to look at the science of ecology. This term was first coined for the study of organisms' interactions with themselves and their environment. It may seem contradictory, at first, but the human host may suffer the most when C.a. is being killed en masse. While this parasite is thriving, its waste products are affecting the host to some extent. But when large numbers of these cells are being destroyed, clearly even more waste products will be released — the entire cell contents, in fact. So the greatest amount of toxins may be released during this period of die-off. Colonics may be recommended to flush out C.a. before antifungals are given in order to reduce the number of organisms and thus the die-off.

The die-off effect is also called the *"HERXHEIMER REACTION"* after the German physician who noted, in the 1920's that during anti-Syphilis treatment with mercury, the worst symptoms occurred shortly after treatment began. This effect may thus occur as any foreign overgrowth is killed in large numbers. The die-off effect for C.a. may last for days or weeks. Curiously, after the Candida Energy Balance, this effect is often mitigated. On the other hand, those with weak immune systems may have a bad die-off as the energy balancing may strengthen the immune system (at last) and it can now "go after" the yeast. (Further energy balancing may obviate this too.) The greater the overgrowth is, the worse the die-off may be. Whatever symptoms existed, before anti-Candida treatment, may be exacerbated during treatment.

Let's return to hypoglycemia. Certain foods (already described) feed the yeast or stress the immune system allowing temporary rapid growth of C.a. Now in their own ecological niche, when the food runs out or internal competition exerts itself, some fungal cells will begin to die off on their own. Thus a Herxheimer-type reaction can occur from ecological forces, we hypothesize. Thus, a few hours after eating a sweet or yeast food, yeast toxins (from excessive growth or die-off) may affect the pancreas leading to hypoglycemia! Thus Candidaisis, in addition to allergies, may possibly cause low or high blood sugar reactions. This is why the term, "**HAC**," (hypoglycemia, allergies, Candida) is used throughout this book.

We note that Candida toxins weaken the immune system and many holistic physicians believe they may play a causative role in immune disorders including allergies, cancer, auto-immune disorders — like lupus — where the body's antibodies attack its own tissues, and perhaps even immune deficiency diseases too. On this author's last lecture tour to Australia, a fascinating report was seen in a health journal. An AIDS victim, near death was brought back to apparently excellent health by antifungal treatment and diet change. We have seen several people recover from Herpes after Candida Energy Balancing. These facts seem to indicate that Candida, or its toxins, weaken the immune system which then allows other germs to take advantage and wreak their own havoc. Of course, the immune system may have been weak in the first place, which allowed Candida to overgrow. Now we're ready to learn about Candida itself.

THE NATURE OF CANDIDA ALBICANS

First we should ask, why is it that this particular fungus — and not others — causes so much trouble in humans? Other families of fungus include Penicillium, Aspergillus, etc. Then in the genus, Candida, there are 70 other species, e.g. Candida tropicalis. Though some of these other fungi may occasionally cause problems in humans, C.a. is the one causing chronic illness in epidemic proportions today. One reason may be that C.a. has protein markers on its cell membrane or wall which are closer to human cell markers than other germs. Recall that a cell's outer covering contains sequences of proteins that our antibodies recognize as foreign, and use as a master template to mass-produce antibodies. See Fig. 1 again. So C.a., with its human-like sequences of markers, may trick the immune system (to some extent) into leaving it alone. In fact, when large numbers of anti-C.a. antibodies are formed, these same antibodies may attack some human tissues as well. (This is an example of auto-immune disease.) These attacked human cells have been found to include thyroid, ovarian and T-Helper (immune) cells. Thus endocrine, female and immune disorders may unfold from this mechanism. For completeness, we note that the one species, C.a., may contain millions of different strains, due to permutations of cell wall marker proteins.

If you have a Candida problem, it would be a good idea to also be tested for allergy to other molds. Some people are helped by neutralization injections for Candida and other molds. Then again, we have spoken to many who got worse from such shots or the preservatives they contain. Maybe one day the ecologists will have the best of both worlds — the potential to offer such shots and the ability to accurately test their allergenicity or toxicity without first injecting them. Yes, we mean simple, rapid, safe muscle testing as described in this book.

Let's return to Candida's toxins now. Candida may produce carbon monoxide; just as its large distant cousin, the mushroom, does. Levine believes that he found the reason some mushroom growers have died after staying in their enclosed areas for long periods of time. It was carbon monoxide poisoning from the mushrooms. Another yeast by-product is *alcohol.* In recent years, in Japan, numerous people have been fired from their jobs for drunkenness. Yet these people swore they never touched alcohol. Blood tests confirmed the charges, however. Physicians believe that C.a. is at fault again. They believe that a new Japanese strain of C.a. secretes more alcohol than acetaldehyde, unlike most previously known strains. They suspect that the American Atomic Bombs dropped in 1945 caused C.a.

to *mutate*. People with overgrowths of this strain only need to eat pasta or ice cream and their yeast will get them drunk! (This makes one wonder about food irradiation. No one is talking about new strains of germs that could result!) The drug Tagamet® has also been shown to lead to overgrowth of the alcohol-producing strain.

Yeast cells apparently also produce steroid, hormone-like substances. They appear to be particularly estrogen-like. Thus, endocrine and sexual disorders can result here. This was suspected for some time as yeast were known to have steroid receptors. The estrogen nature of the yeast "hormones" is said to cause the enlarged breasts found in some heavy beer drinkers. Analogously, some researchers believe that some women with very small breasts may have had a Candida problem during their puberty years. So, in women with large breasts, a Candida problem *may not* have been a life long problem. There is also a genetic component here. Now as we all have some intestinal yeast and yeast secretes hormone-like substances, it may be that our endocrine systems have evolved to co-exist and interact with the expected small amounts of these substances. After all, we depend on the acidophilus bacteria for some of its products. Higher life forms could only evolve along with the already existing lower forms. It is speculative, but perhaps some symbiosis-like effect was meant to occur if C.a. exists in appropriately small amounts in the colon.

Now C.a. is said to be a dimorphic fungus — it has two major forms. In the yeast budding form, it is said to be less invasive locally. (But as it is smaller and less "attached," it may be able to migrate more in this form?) In the invasive form, C.a. grows mycelia — branch- or thread-like structures that can dig into human cells and extract nutrients. This can be one cause of a permeable GI tract, which we have noted can help lead to allergies.

We have seen recent micrographs of 8 forms of C.a.; therefore, much is yet to be learned about this organism. It is speculated that Candida albicans can occur in a very small state and enter the cell and perhaps even the nucleus. If it enters the nucleus, it may be able to alter the genetic material.

Some say that Candida albicans, like other fungi, can exist in a spore-like state. In this semi-hibernating form, it may be much more difficult to kill. In its more usual forms, Candida albicans not only ingests sugar, but uses this molecule as the building block for the fibers it makes to attach to its hosts tissues. (Another reason to cut down on sweets.) In a related matter, some reports indicate that intravenous glucose drips, can contribute to yeast overgrowth in the blood. Let us now examine various substances used to combat Candida.

ANTIFUNGAL AGENTS

1. Iodine
2. Gentian Violet
3. Nystatin
4. Ketoconazole
5. Amphotericin-B
6. Diflucan
7. Garlic (Allicin)
8. Pau D'Arco
9. Australian Tea Tree Oil
10. Other herbs including cloves and echinecea
11. Caprylic Acid
12. Acidic substances like sorbic acid, lactic acid
13. Oxygenators: ozone, hydrogen peroxide, chlorine dioxide
14. Selenium
15. Magnesium
16. Germanium
17. Acidophilus (see below). Overgrowths of Candida and parasites should be eliminated *first* as acidophilus bacteria often feed—*not* displace—Candida or Protozoan parasites, which are heartier.

Let's look first at the more medical substances. Iodine may have been one of the first antifungal drugs used. Next Gentian Violet was used. Nurses coated the tongues of newborns (with thrush) with this substance. The newborn may have picked up the yeast as it passed through its mother's vagina. Gentian Violet is freely available in some countries, like Australia, but a prescription is needed in the U.S.

Most of the first books about Candidiasis recommended *NYSTATIN* as "the drug of choice." Its name indicates where it was discovered — growing in milk on a dairy farm in New York State. It is actually a mold derivative. Thus it can be allergenic. Also, the preferred, excipient-free, powder has been occasionally produced in "bad batches." These may preferentially get shipped overseas. These batches are not quite what they should be, they may be somewhat altered and toxic. Quality control has supposedly been improved now, to meet the increased demand.

Nystatin works by destroying Candida's cell wall. It is most effective in the GI tract because it is poorly absorbed into the blood. Thus it is said to have little kidney or liver toxicity, as the other, newer drugs may. But, if a systemic problem does exist, Nystatin may be ineffective for the same reason. Huge doses would be needed for systemic Candidiasis. In patients with leukemia and Candida septicemia, up to 60 tablets a day have been used, to keep the yeast from literally taking over its immuno-compromised host. Despite all the "magic bullet" claims of the first books, we have seen that many with E.I. do not seem to get well even after years of taking it. (Of course, those that did get well from such therapy may not be reading this book.) Some medical researchers, using the controversial live-cell microscopy technique, claim Nystatin just causes C.a. to mutate into a cell wall-free form. Then it is said to be smaller and able to get into the blood and migrate. Other researchers deny this. All this researcher can say is that we have taught the HEBS methods around the world, and many cities seem to have their Candida support groups comprised of people who tried this drug for years? There are no magic bullets. Even the energy balancing alone (without diet and other restrictions) will usually not do the trick.

More potent and systemic drugs exist. In the U.S., *KETOCONAZOLE* is the next "drug of choice." This medication interferes with C.a.'s steroid receptors, which will destroy the cell membrane. The hypothesized Nystatin-induced mutation is said not to occur from Ketoconazole. This drug is absorbed into the blood—more efficiently than the other two drugs. Thus it can be systemically effective but it also has kidney and liver toxicity. The patient's blood levels need to be monitored frequently. In its first year of use, a small but significant number of people died. But this is no longer seen as a problem as smaller doses and better monitoring were realized. Not legal in the U.S., but used often in Britain and Australia is Amphotericin-B. Its said to be even more potent than Ketoconazole and to work similarly. And these two are synthetic drugs, not mold derivatives.

Some herbs and foods have long been known to have antifungal properties. They may be less potent and much less toxic. Garlic may be the oldest such food. Allicin is the purported antifungal and antibacterial agent in garlic. Onions may have similar properties to a much lesser extent. Which garlic supplements are effective is also hotly and legally debated. You can always eat the raw stuff too! Cooking may destroy the allicin as may the processes used in making a supplement.

The tree bark variously known as *PAU D'ARCO*, La Pacho, Taheebo, or Ipe Roxo grows in the Amazon regions of Brazil and Argentina. Most trees in the high humidity, and thus moldy air, of the Amazons succumb to the air-borne fungus. But not so, this one species. The local Indians have used this bark for everything from stomach aches to cancer. Brazilian medical researchers are now studying it for similar purposes. It is also alkalinizing. Always remember, anything taken too often can become allergenic too.

Australia's Tea Tree Oil is said to be one of the most potent antifungals, even against the spores. It is used on fungal skin and nails. Internally, only a drop or two is recommended. We're told if diluted with aloe vera, larger doses can be used. This oil, which smells like turpentine, is now readily available in the U.S. We believe, it may be contra-recommended for those with Epstein-Barr Virus, as it may contain the class of chemicals that reactivate the virus. There are many other herbs known to have some antifungal properties, including cloves and echinecea. Other herbs, some experts say, are needed to strengthen the liver in Candida patients.[B]

Caprylic acid is a short chain fatty acid derived from coconuts that has been much used lately for Candidiasis. It is said to coat the gastrointestinal tract and help starve Candida albicans. We have found nearly all such supplements to be highly allergenic and not well tolerated. Phenols may be used as binders here. Again there is the priceless advantage of using Applied Kinesiology for testing before trying any of these agents.

Some say that overly alkaline intestines (vagina, etc.) can help yeast overgrow. Thus acidic substances are used to counteract the alkalinity. Sorbic acid is available as a mouthwash and douche. Lactic acid, found in cabbage juice, is also used. Some gynecologists recommend vinegar for its acid nature. But they are apparently unaware of the molds in the vinegar. We do not recommend vinegar.

Next we come to the acidophilus bacteria. Please first see our warning at the bottom of page 85.   Reimplanting the gut's friendly flora — the acidophilus bacteria — may be necessary to prevent or overcome yeast overgrowth. The same may be true for vaginal problems. Several caveats here. There are many different strains of acidophilus. Some are effective and others are not. Then too, many supplement companies sell worthless products! The acidophilus may be a weak strain or it may have been killed in the manufacturing or shipping process. Many people take acidophilus for years without re-establishing them — often because parasites or Candida eat them! The best acidophilus is shipped via rapid air delivery and needs to be refrigerated. Besides acidophilus, other friendly flora include Bifidus, Bulgaricus, and Streptococcus faecium.

Mercury, as from dental fillings, may also prevent this needed regrowth. Because of allergy, yoghurt and milk containing acidophilus is usually contraindicated. Soy based yoghurt is now available in health food stores. It is also possible to overdo supplementation of these and other bacterial species with resultant overgrowth and GI complaints. Yes, it's complicated. MBT can actually help *before* you try something, but what is happening to your body will always be the most accurate gauge! If you get ill from some antifungal agent, advanced MBT can help determine if a die-off, allergy or toxicity is involved. Even potential effectiveness can be individually tested! Those with Candidiasis need all the help, without being harmed, that they can get!

Biotin is another nutrient recommended to hold the yeast in check. It is said to prevent mycelia growth. But excesses can feed the yeast as noted here. Interestingly, some kinesiologists, using advanced methods find avoidance of all B-vitamins is needed for some[22] until the yeast problem is eliminated. This is in contradistinction to many nutritionists' recommendations. They also believe iron, zinc, and possibly even acidophilus may favor yeast overgrowth. Only MBT seems to offer such a truly individualized approach. Yet some with E.I. may need these nutrients to strengthen their immune system. Again diagnostic tests and MBT needs to be done on an individual basis.

Various agents are purported to kill fungus and other germs via *OXYGENATION*. These include hydrogen peroxide, ozone, and stabilized aqueous chlorine dioxide (Purogene, Dioxychlor, Alcide). Ozone machines can ozonate water, the colon and can even be used intravenously. Peroxide can be added to water or used intravenously. Some nutritionists warn against peroxide because of free radical damage, not just to the yeast, but to the host's immune system as well. We tend to favor this view, but have also heard positive feedback. We have seen some good results with the Purogene mouthwash and skin cream.

Perhaps the two most important minerals for fighting Candida are *SELENIUM* and *MAGNESIUM*. Studies have shown that macrophages (killer white blood cells) can surround Candida albicans, but can't secrete their deadly enzymes if they're low on selenium. They will eventually let go. Magnesium has been found to be crucial in the restoration of metabolic and immunologic competence in those with Candidiasis. Older nutritional dogma recommended calcium to magnesium supplementation in the ratio of 2 to 1. This has often proven harmful to the E.I. They need at least as much magnesium as calcium and frequently more! Specific agents also counteract Candida's main toxin, acetaldehyde.

ANTI-ACETALDEHYDE NUTRIENTS
1. Vitamin C
2. Vitamin B$_1$ (Thiamine)
3. Vitamin B$_5$ (Pantothenic Acid)
4. Taurine (an amino acid)
5. Cysteine (an amino acid)
6. *Molybdenum*[23] Perhaps this mineral is most crucial of all.

These nutrients are also anti-formaldehyde agents. (The spider plant also absorbs environmental formaldehyde.) The chapter on nutrition will detail the anti-oxidant nutrients which the immune system needs. We will also shortly examine the crucial HEBS energy balancing methods. This is the first book to detail this essential, additional dimension.

Lastly, we wish to inform you of the immense power of the advanced H.E.B.S. kinesiology methods as regards Candida and Parasite Balancing. With these advanced methods, we can actually determine what herbs, nutrients or even a physician's drugs would be effective against *that person's* Candida (or Parasite) problem *at that time*. We would then use our kinesiology methods to see if these agents were toxic or allergic at that time. Here is the holy grail of all health and medicine. We can determine—before the person takes the remedy—if it would be both safe and effective! Truly, the healer of the *21st Century* has arrived! Months or years of expensive and possibly harmful hit-and-miss or trial-and-error attempts to eradicate overgrowths can thus be avoided. Of course, *practitioners are often trying to eliminate overgrowths of "critters" that aren't even there.* This includes, quite frequently, attempting to kill Candida overgrowths when it is really Protozoan parasites that are present. (Candida may have already been eliminated, leaving the Protozoan parasites which are untouched by antifungal agents, or Candida overgrowth was never really present.)

Our advanced HEBS methods are first used to immediately determine the imbalance and thus which "critters" are actually likely to be present. Someone personally *certified* by this author (as determined by contacting us directly) with the advanced HEBS methods can do this and may also recommend an end to taking a previous "remedy" if ineffectiveness, toxicity or allergenicity is found. Perhaps one day, all physicians and practitioners will learn these methods (as the medical physician who wrote our foreword recommends) and observe the remarkable and rapid results.

8

Epstein-Barr—Chronic Fatigue—Virus, Fibromyalgia, Cryptocides, Parasites, and Symbiosis

Here we will describe other infectious agents that have been found to play a large role in chronic (or ecological) illness. They are often undiagnosed or misdiagnosed or considered "subclinical." They may occur subsequent to Candidiasis (or Parasitosis) or independently of it.

EPSTEIN-BARR AND OTHER VIRUSES

Just as with Protozoan parasites (below), chronic, low-level infections of viruses are now seen as frequent components of Ecological Illness. The most notorious "ecological virus" is the *EPSTEIN-BARR VIRUS*. The chronic condition due to this germ is known as Chronic Epstein-Barr Virus or **CEBV**. (It's also been called **"CHRONIC FATIGUE SYNDROME"** and "yuppie disease.")

A more recent term is **FIBROMYALGIA** whose sufferers also have fatigue, aches and pains. A fascinating aside about fibromyalgia. The chart of its "never-to-touch pain points" coincides with the kinesiologist's neurolymphatic points which should be rubbed to re-set them—*and lead to wellness*—and they will hurt (everyone). This author's research revealed that *despite all these different names, Parasitosis (the earliest cause), Candidiasis, allergies (and addictions) and blood sugar disorders are common to all of these maladies and all our eminently curable with our methods!* The Epstein-Barr virus also causes mononucleosis (a.k.a. mono or "kissing disease"). In the 1980's, physicians found a non-acute, chronic syndrome caused by the same virus. There will be no enlarged liver or spleen or month-long, near-paralysis as in the acute form.

SYMPTOMS OF CHRONIC EPSTEIN-BARR VIRUS

1. Fatigue, Fibromyalgia
2. Depression (hormones and neurotransmitters are interfered with by the virus or other microorganisms present)
3. Muscle aches and pain
4. Headaches
5. Severe chemical sensitivities and/or electromagnetic sensitivities
6. Swollen lymph glands
7. "Frequent colds"
8. Throat pain
9. Most CEBV sufferers have Parasitosis (the initial cause), Allergies, Candidiasis and Hypoglycemia if tested

We follow up on #9 above, first. We believe CEBV has been overplayed in the media and Parasitosis, hypoglycemia, allergies and Candidiasis (PHAC) underplayed. Many CEBV sufferers go to the "CEBV Expert" for supplements and other help. These "experts" often know little about the PHAC syndrome. Often allergic supplements are used. The "CEBV patient" often doesn't progress far after spending much time and money with the expert. We've seen many people recently who thought their fatigue was CEBV only to have Parasitosis, hypoglycemia, allergies or Candidiasis or some combination revealed as the cause of their complaints. Others, of course, have all four.

Now let's return to other symptoms listed above. Fatigue is perhaps the most common complaint people have. It can be caused by hundreds of maladies, including Parasitosis, hypoglycemia, allergies and Candidiasis. So how can you tell "what is causing what?" There are several ways. One way of uncovering the cause(s) of your problems was described in Chapter 4. This was *by the type of foods craved.*

A second factor is the type of allergies you have. Universal (food, chemical and pollen) allergy is linked to Parasitosis or Candidiasis; these weaken the immune system leading to CEBV. The key with Candida is actually pollen allergies. This is because chemical and electromagnetic allergies can be tied to CEBV (or other viruses) and food allergies occur from gastrointestinal permeability and/or from overeating foods. Hidden Parasitosis is often the earliest factor leading to a chronic viral condition.

Medical tests (see Appendix B) and distinguishing symptoms are two additional factors used to eliminate different possibilities. For these, you need a physician. But you can determine the types of allergies and cravings you have on your own—once you realize their nature.

Now for Epstein-Barr Virus, "chemical sensitivities" takes on an even more insidious nature. The ubiquitous *TUNG OILS* (found in everything from paint to furniture polish) are one relevant class of chemicals here. These chemicals don't just initiate an allergy, per se, they can actually *re-activate* the virus—which may have been dormant! The viruses then replicate en masse. This author wonders whether this virus might not be lying dormant in everyone. Perhaps its chronic form would be unknown, were it not for the sad state of the modern environment?! Recall the Ecologically Ill are more permeable to the external environment. That is, only in those whose bodies allow Tung Oils to enter the blood, can the EBV get a chance to reactivate. Note, celery may naturally contain a high amount of viruses and should be muscle-tested for allergy.

We in HEBS have always perceived that avoiding the 20th Century is an impossibility and realized that the body could be strengthened more naturally. Energy balancing for CEBV has proven effective in many people where diet, supplementation and avoidance produced little improvement.

But first, accurate testing is needed. Most physicians, to humor their patient, would perform the usual test for the Epstein-Barr virus. But this looks only for the one antibody related to the acute form—mononucleosis—and *not* for the chronic form. Better diagnostic labs look for elevated levels of three or four different antibodies. This testing can even determine if a past, chronic or acute case was once present.

I can recall, in my first year of graduate Physics study, getting very ill with a virus. I was laid up in bed for a week. But after this I suffered from constant throat pain and my fatigue was markedly increased. (The infirmary physicians [pediatricians] at SUNY at Stony Brook just prescribed their modern snake oil—Valium®.) Looking back at my entire life, I am sure I had allergy and Candida and Parasite problems; but this viral syndrome (totally unknown at the time) was "the beginning of the end." After this I finally developed bad hay fever and within a few years was fighting for my life as detailed in the introduction. I had swollen glands and frequent "viruses" for years afterwards. The CEBV as well as the Candidiasis was taken care of, after the 1983 "Candida Balance!" But I had the full E-B Virus antibody panel-test afterwards. Sure enough, the interpretation said "evidence of past chronic EBV, but no present problem. (I never had "mono".) No doubt Parasitosis, Allergies, Candidiasis and a weak immune system led to my CEBV. But once this occurred, illness unfolded even more rapidly. Candida can predispose to CEBV, but the reverse is true. We've seen some people that apparently picked up the Epstein-Barr Virus first. Totally inappropriate antibiotic therapy then led to Candidiasis.

Australia and New Zealand have seen the rise of a devastating illness called M.E. (Myalgic Encephalomyeltis) or Post Viral Syndrome. Here the muscle fatiguing and wasting is so pronounced that some sufferers have had their bones break! One researcher believes that the related virus, the *Coxsackie Virus,* is the cause. But all the components of P.H.A.C. are involved. On one of my lecture tours to these two countries, I was pleased to see how much HEBS was able to help these lovely people. We saw some immediate and dramatic improvements right in the seminar! One fellow couldn't even fold his arms until the Rochlitz Heart-Integration™ was performed. (See Chapter 11.) Then he had no trouble. Blood pressure was normalized in others. And you can't have allergy to energy balancing!

Besides CEBV and the Coxsackie virus, *Cytomegalovirus* (**CMV**) and *Herpes* may play a role in some cases of E.I. Many of these viruses are found in AIDS patients, who like the E.I. have weak immune systems. But don't worry, statistically most with E.I. have little incidence of AIDS or even Cancer. A different etiology is apparently present. The *Physicist's Rapid Solution* involves, as always, energy balancing *in addition* to nutrition and avoidance. These viruses, like Candida and parasites, may be present in small amounts in all of us.

We need to prevent or overcome the overgrowths. We've seen several people that were helped by the advanced Parasite or Candida Balance intrinsically, but some needed specific energy balancing for EBV. Again, this is not a medical treatment for a disease. Rather it patches up energy blockages that can then hopefully allow the body's natural defenses to do the job.

Recently, we have researched the use of electrical "zappers." These little electrical devices impart, at the wrist area, small electrical currents of the appropriate frequency to kill viruses. We have found them effective against cold viruses and chemical sensitivity-causing viruses. The original research, done at Albert Einstein Medical College in New York showed certain frequencies killed the AIDS Virus quite well. Then "Big Brother" forcibly ended the research! Some people also claim great weight loss after zapper use. Some also claim the zappers can kill all "critters" including parasites. We think it can only kill weaker organisms; namely the viruses, as the original medical research demonstrated. The zapper we tested and found effective is now available from our headquarters by contacting us as noted at the end of this book.

There are nutrients that can help the body fight viruses too. These include Vitamins A and C and the amino acid lysine and the compound lauric acid. Also highly touted are special egg lecithin extracts with the 7 to 2 to 1 (7:2:1) ratio of lecithin components. These lecithin extracts were first found by Israeli researchers to help prevent the AIDS virus from getting through the cell membrane. Anti-viral agents are listed below.

ANTI-VIRAL AGENTS
Egg Lecithin Extracts (7:2:1) ratio
Vitamin A
Vitamin C
Lysine (an amino acid)
Lauric Acid
Zinc
Garlic
"Zappers"

PROGENITOR CRYPTOCIDES

Now let's discuss the remarkable germ Progenitor Cryptocides[24] (**P.C.**). [It is pronounced Pro-gen-i-tor Cryp-toe-cide-ees.] Most of the research done on this germ was performed by Virginia Livingston(-Wheeler), M.D. (now deceased). She believed P.C. is "*the* cancer causing germ." P.C. is rigorously a bacterium. But its name is derived from the fact that it can change size and shape and form. It can supposedly shrink down to viral size and possibly enter the cell and/or nucleus. And it can exist as a larger spore-like entity too.

P.C. can exist in an innocuous form or in a "*virulent*, cancer-causing form." Livingston believed that nearly all chicken contains P.C. in the cancer-causing form! (Yes, it would be in the egg too. This is the age old question: which will kill you first, the chicken or the egg?) Apparently other fowl may not be a problem. Chickens are forced to mature at a very rapid rate through the use of artificial hormones. (This is not the case for so-called free-range chicken or their eggs.) It is equivalent to forcing a human to mature in six months, instead of 18 years! We note that many have cut down on red meat and eat much chicken. If one is cancer-prone, Livingston would caution against this. Of course, unless organic, all American meats contain hormones, antibiotics, tranquilizers and other chemicals.

In her San Diego clinic, Livingston treated cancer patients with diet, nutrition (including a Vitamin A derivative) and her attenuated Cryptocides vaccine. She reported an 80% cure rate during the last 20 years. Most of her patients already had their immune systems compromised via orthodox treatment with chemotherapy and radiation! (Holistic means sadly are often the last, and not the first, methods tried.) For her remarkable work, Livingston received scorn and persecution instead of the Nobel Prize she deserved.

Livingston also shipped dry-ice packed chickens that were inoculated with her vaccine. (It might be less expensive to just forego chicken.) Despite the claims of organic chicken farmers, she believed this is the only way to guarantee P.C.-free chicken. We refer again to the virulent form of P.C. Her vaccine has come to be accepted in agricultural circles as an effective anti-tumor agent in chickens. Livingston attempted to prove her work to mainstream "cancer specialists." Billions of dollars are spent looking for mythical viruses by these "experts." We note that clinical ecologists might speculate that parasites or Candida plays a role in cancer too. We might hypothesize that these stronger microbes weaken the immune system first. After all, not everyone who eats chicken will get cancer. There are, of course, many other additional factors involved in cancer.

In 1974, Livingston made the remarkable discovery that P.C. is carried by human sperm and secretes a hormone that is essential for fertilization and for the fetus to grow and survive! This hormone, choriogonadotropin (**CG**), apparently enables fetal cells to grow and multiply and protects them from the mother's immune system. Thus, P.C. is necessary for all human life to start! When the immune system is weakened, P.C. may come out of its dormancy and again secrete CG, also called Human CG or HCG, hormone. Without a fetus to utilize it, it may now lead to tumor growth. So, as with Candida, everyone has P.C. within them, only *overgrowths* or sudden changes in P.C.'s *virulence* causes a problem.

We speculate that the *THYROID* plays a key role in Cryptocides effects on both humans and chickens. Medical researchers are known to use chickens to mimic human thyroid disorders— thyroiditis. And some holistic physicians note that Cancer patients have a history of thyroid problems. (We also note that many Cancer patients have an earlier history of fungal nails, thrush, etc.) Energy testing indicates P.C. may affect the thyroid and that Candida or Parasite imbalance may have occurred first. P.C. may secrete acetaldehyde or other fungal product, if it can exist in a fungal, or even spore-like state. (Bacteria ordinarily are known not to secrete acetaldehyde.) If so, brain and heart integration can be affected. (See the chapters on these affects.)

Finally, we note that a Cryptocides allergy may exist. After all, Bacterial allergy *is* known. And allergists have treated women who were severely allergic to their spouse's semen. It is possible this germ or the HCG hormone was the allergenic component. In these rare cases, vaginal or oral introduction of semen led to anaphylactic reactions! But it is impossible to know, for certain, just what in the semen is causing the reaction.

PARASITES—*THE EARLIEST CAUSE*

Parasites can include any opportunistic organism growing in or on its human host, to the detriment of the host. (Candida albicans, bacteria, viruses, etc. would be included.) Here, however, we will discuss one-celled Protozoans and worms. As we have noted, a weakened immune system, or digestive system, can allow overgrowths of these organisms in the first place. We believe that the ultimate cause of ecological illness, chronic fatigue syndrome and fibromyalgia may—for many—be the lack of breast-feeding in infancy. This creates a lifetime of low immunity and gastrointestinal weakness that will often make parasitosis or Candidiasis inevitable. A fragile potassium metabolism, this author believes, is also often involved. (Our special advanced kinesiology testing indicates this.) We have found this to be most prevalent in those that have an Eastern European lineage. But anyone can get a shock to the immune system which can possibly lead to parasitosis. Also, if the host has diminished stomach hydrochloric acid and/or pancreatic enzymes, parasites may take hold. These substances not only digest food, they also digest any ingested germs. But this is a vicious cycle as Protozoan parasitosis often causes the stomach to shut down production of pepsin and hydrochloric acid.

Let's look at the two *ONE-CELLED PROTOZOANS: Entamoeba histolytica* (an amoeba) and *Giardia lamblia*. These may be *the ultimate causes of ecological illness, chronic fatigue and fibromyalgia.* They weaken the immune system allowing for Candida, Epstein-Barr Virus, etc. to then take hold. In the GI tract, they can absorb the host's nutrients and make the intestines *permeable*. The latter effect, we believe, occurs because the parasites—especially the amoeba—interfere with potassium metabolism. Recall that permeability can lead to allergies as undigested food may enter the blood. From the GI tract, parasites, or their toxins, may move to other organs. Giardia, e.g., may gravitate to the *gall bladder*. So it may be possible for distant organs to be affected by parasites or their waste products, if the latter gets into the blood. The liver, pancreas (blood sugar and digestive enzyme problems), adrenals (fatigue or anxiety states) and brain are usually adversely affected by parasite toxins. We have found that slightly raised (blood-colored) red spots on the (abdominal) skin and enlarged pupils often indicate parasitosis. The crucial inhibitory neurotransmitter serotonin is often severely adversely affected. Most of the serotonergic nerves are actually in the GI tract! This can then lead to severe depression, great anxiety, even paranoia and schizophrenia.

So parasites may actually be the primary cause of much chronic illness. Any symptom (including all those listed in this book) attributed to Candida, may actually be due to one or both of these Protozoans, which over 80% of Candidiasis sufferers are known to harbor. The hidden amoebiasis, in particular, can cause grave, immediate and universal food allergies. Rotating any remaining safe foods may be a necessity for survival until the parasites are killed and the extreme permeability thus terminated. The clinical ecologists' neutralizations are thus seen as a waste of time and money and they usually become allergenic themselves too! Parasites, especially the amoeba, interfere with potassium and make the intestines permeable—hence the allergies and a weak immune system. *Killing 100% of the parasites—with our advanced methods—and performing our energy balancing will usually completely terminate ecological illness, chronic fatigue and fibromyalgia!* Indeed, with our advanced methods, the die-off percentage can even be monitored. 100% must be reached or they grow back.

All stool culture tests—including the one used by many holistic physicians—*virtually never* find the amoeba or giradia! The parasites attach to the GI tract and will not be expelled in the stool. The test by Louis Parish, M.D., the *rectal smear test* involves placing a hollow tube in the rectum, and through this, a probe nicks the intestinal wall for a minute. The sample is then observed under a special microscope. The parasites are then seen and classified. Only this and our advanced kinesiology, are accurate tests. Advanced HEBS kinesiology can even indicate what remedies are effective and non-allergenic before taking them! This can save months or even years of the usual guesswork! The stressful die-off effect is also mitigated by the HEBS methods.

Giardiasis may be a rampant problem in the U.S. today. Over

50% of the water supply is contaminated with it and (unlike bacteria) it's not killed by chlorination. Raw, organic fruits and vegetables are often a tremendous source of giardias and amoebas!! Organic usually means that the produce was fertilized with what comes out of the rear ends of horses and cows. But, this is the focal point of the giardias and amoebas!! Much produce goes to industrialized nations from third world countries where the animal dung is again the fertilizer. Pesticide-free produce is great, but *cook it* to kill the Protozoans. Eat only cooked foods!! Food handlers in restaurants are known to transmit these protozoans too. Pets and improperly cooked meats are other sources. Most with E.I. are being found to have one or both of the giardia or amoeba, even though many have never been to a "tropical country." Amoebiasis is also linked to rheumatoid arthritis, gum, vaginal and skin (psoriasis) problems. The Protozoan parasite, *Cryptocides* is often found in water too. *Cyclospora* occurs frequently on fruits from tropical countries.

Physicians in the U.S. almost never address the issue of larger parasites — *WORMS*. However, in some European countries, people de-worm themselves along with their pets every six months. One needn't be emaciated to harbor worms or Protozoan parasites. The rectal smear or stool culture tests should ascertain the presence of worms, or more likely their ova or eggs.

Killing worms can be complicated. Naturopaths and holistic M.D.'s often have vivid or gruesome stories in this regard. It is difficult to get all of a worm. Agents that expel or kill worms often don't get the heads of these segmented creatures. The head probably has a good grip on its host and doesn't want to leave. One natural remedy has been to sit in a tub of goat's milk and take herbs or medication to expel the head. With the delicious goat's milk waiting, the head may leave, but often a "helpful hand" is needed. We've also been told of this last method being used orally too! But drugs or herbs can nowadays do the job.

Be careful when taking anti-parasitic drugs. Usually, ten day trials are the maximum period allowed for Flagyl®. Blood monitoring may be needed to prevent liver damage. Yodoxin® (20-day trial) is the only drug that can kill the cysts of the *Entamoeba histolytica.*

There are many natural and effective remedies available for these purposes too. Issue #2 of the HEBS Newsletter, *The Human Ecology Balancing Scientist* lists various herbs and nutrients effective against parasites. [Energy balancing is also noted in the above article. —see the back of this book.] These remedies include garlic, Black Walnut leaves, dry papaya seeds, seaweed, homeopathic dilutions of Ipecac, aloe vera, Echinecea, and Russian Black Radish. Other more recent agents being used include Para-Stat (*Holarrhena antidysenterica* and Indrajae), Biocidin, and AP Mag. Take nothing in alcohol! Citrus seed extract may be able to kill Candida, but it is too feeble to kill the protozoans or their (protective) cyst-states. We recommend against taking the herb, *Artemesia annua* (form of wormwood) unless our advanced kinesiology tests are used. While it may kill parasites (and their cysts) in some, it can also drastically interfere with potassium in others (as the parasites may already be doing.) People of Eastern European ethnicity are likely to have this potassium problem from Artemesia annua. *It can be lethal if one gets a severe potassium interference problem from Artemesia annua.*

Once the intestines no longer function up to par, many types of germs may overgrow. Always see if you can ascertain the cause or source of parasites. Is it water (get a good filter—see the back of the book), raw produce, or pets? We're always amazed to see people kissing their pets after the pets have been in the street doing things we can't describe here. Cats are known to harbor Toxoplasma, Candida and other organisms. Also cooking meats properly is essential. Raw or undercooked meat or fish can be the source of worms and protozoans. Advanced energy balancing can harmonize and strengthen the body in specific regard to any of the organisms noted here. This non-medical method is safe and natural.

SYMBIOSIS

As you might expect, someone with a weak immune system may simultaneously harbor overgrowths of several of the germs noted in this chapter. Symbiosis is the biological term for the mutual occupation of a niche by two (or more) different organisms. Each may produce substances that the other needs to survive.

A graphic symbiosis in some with E.I. was found by microbiologist Eunice Carlson, Ph.D. If you recall, *Toxic Shock Syndrome* (TSS), made many women ill, and even led to numerous deaths in the 70's, until Carlson found the culprit. It was overgrowths of the Staphylococcus aureus bacterium in women who used certain tampons. Tampon design was subsequently changed. But several years later, Carlson found that TSS occurred *only* in women with chronic vaginal Candidiasis! She has taken very vivid micrographs of the symbiosis of the Staph bacterium and C.a. thriving together. If the yeast cells surround the Staph cells, the immune system can't get at the latter. Carlson's studies revealed that healthy women could have *one million* Staph germs implanted vaginally without developing TSS. But, in women with Candidiasis, only *five* bacteria were needed to lead to TSS! Thus we see how further illness can unfold if an overgrowth of one germ (and/or a weak immune system) exists.

Some holistic physicians believe that C.a. can become symbiotic with a host of other organisms. These include other fungi, e.g., *Mucor racemosus* (which is present in organic compost), clostridium, penicillium, and aspergillus. Also chlamydia, a bacterium-like organism, may be symbiotic with the yeast. Other possible symbiants could include parasites, viruses and Cryptocides. Indeed, we can speculate that symbiosis may be present in many with long term E.I.! Unilateral disease states may be a simplistic approximation. (Physicists too, at first, make simple models of natural phenomenon, but do let go when the evidence shows itself.)

In HEBS, we have extended symbiosis to the term "effective symbiosis." Now, we know from studies of human behavior, that when one smells a familiar smell, a simultaneous visual recall often occurs too (or vice versa). Thus several senses can be incorporated, via associated neural firing patterns, into one memory state. Analogously, we believe that two or more simultaneously occurring energy imbalances can become incorporated into one "symbiotic imbalance." So it is possible that any continuous, or continual, detrimental, environmental, ecological and even emotional imbalance can become "symbiotic" with Candida imbalance. These symbiotic factors could thus include other organisms, any type of allergy, emotions, etc. Advanced HEBS procedures include the "Anti-Symbiotic Balance" to restore balance if two, or more negative synergists have simultaneously weakened the body's energies. Just as physicians would hopefully, simultaneously treat both the yeast and the Staph in women with TSS. Treating (or balancing) one's overgrowth (or energy imbalance) sequentially may not work.

As the TSS symbiosis indicates, the whole can be more than the sum of its parts. Perhaps many ills will someday be viewed as symbioses. This may include AIDS as many organisms may be involved in this illness. C.a. (a germ found in the colon) and Cryptocides (in sperm) may play a role in AIDS, as would parasitosis. But this is speculation and it is difficult to ascertain cause from effect when the immune system is destroyed. (Other researchers hypothesize AIDS is caused by man-made viruses introduced by smallpox and Hepatitis vaccines. Some researchers say the HIV virus has never been proven to cause AIDS.)

Many germs may have some capacity to change size and shape and even genetic material under suitable conditions, as C.a. and P.C. are known to. The *Helicobacter pylori* bacterium may overgrow in the stomach (and maybe elsewhere). It is the germ that often causes bad breath (halitosis), or ulcers of the stomach. We speculate that it may be capable of ulcerating the small and large intestines too, as in ileitis and colitis. It is a potent germ and has even been found in the inner linings of blood vessels and may be causative in cardiovascular degenerative disease!

This germ may be capable of causing permeability as parasites are. It may also be another secondary opportunistic organism overgrowing after Protozoan parasitosis weakens the human host first. Medical physicians use a triple antibiotic containing bismuth to kill the H.p. bacterium. We find that various herbs readily to do the job. One such herb is mastic gum, a resin of the *Pistacia lenticus* tree.

9

MUSCLE BIOFEEDBACK TESTING or KINESIOLOGY

Now we digress from purely ecological matters, to begin our discussion of the other half of the *PHYSICIST'S RAPID SOLUTION*—energy testing and balancing. To test the body for imbalances (including ecological ones), we need some *feedback system* to give us information on the body's current state and its reactions to external stimuli. Biofeedback has become a familiar concept nowadays. Stress management and lie detectors both make use of changes in skin cell electrical conductivity in response to something as "esoteric" as a thought or memory.

George Goodheart, D.C., in the early 1960's discovered that small changes in muscle strength could also be used as a feedback system. Now the study of "kinesiology," per se, had been around for many years. Kinesiology entails placing arms and legs in certain positions which isolate a single muscle. A testor then would ask the subject to resist the testor's push or pull on the arm or leg. It could be determined whether a muscle was functioning properly in this way.

But Goodheart went way beyond this. He found that by stretching muscles in certain ways, he could make weak muscles go strong almost instantly. He also discovered that individual muscles were energetically connected to the body's acupuncture meridian system. And these acupuncture meridians have been known for thousands of years to energize the body's organs. So there exists a feedback system of muscles to acupuncture meridians and from these to the organs. This is the

MUSCLE / MERIDIAN / ORGAN linkage. So by using muscle strength changes as feedback, the state of the related acupuncture meridian (as well as the muscle itself), could be immediately measured. Indirectly, the organ's energy may be gauged by testing its related muscle, too. As the organ's energy may not correlate with any pathological (disease) state, we should advise against misinterpreting muscle testing as "medical" in any way. Licensed physicians can, of course, do precisely this.

Goodheart called his discovery "Applied Kinesiology" and shared his discoveries within the chiropractic profession. In the early 70's, Goodheart formed the International College of Applied Kinesiology (ICAK) which is only open to licensed physicians—primarily chiropractors.

Others went on to share Applied Kinesiology with lay people around the world. This author was fortunate to learn of this new science in 1980. It immediately changed my life, and became an intimate part of my life from then on. Every single person who is chronically ill, has allergies, etc., needs to learn and master this new but simple body of knowledge. It belongs to you, not (just) your doctor! This book was written, in part, with this goal.

Since the first edition came out, countless thousands of people have mastered the kinesiological techniques in this book and finally attained wellness. Though Applied Kinesiology (**A.K.**) was devised by Goodheart, for testing muscle and spinal imbalances, it has been greatly expanded since then. Goodheart's original discovery, and his many later contributions, merit a Nobel Prize in Medicine. The potential value for muscle testing and balancing is limitless! It is used today by chiropractic physicians, medical physicians, dentists, nutritionists, psychologists, massage therapists, educators, vision therapists, a few clinical ecologists, and many others. Even in its most simple form, Applied Kinesiology can gauge imbalance and help restore balance to muscles, meridians, spine, lymph, and circulatory systems.

The key is that many imbalances can be *immediately* tested. Dentists can determine problems in teeth and psychologists can rapidly uncover and correct emotional stress. Variations of A.K. have other names including: muscle response testing, Touch for Health, muscle testing or just kinesiology. Here we use the term *"Muscle Biofeedback Testing"* or MBT because this term more clearly defines what is actually going on. MBT can even be used to quickly ascertain the body's nutritional status. (This should never be used exclusively in place of blood, urine, and hair tests.) Robert Riddler, D.C. found that nutritional deficiencies can be gauged simply by touching certain points on the body and simultaneously performing the MBT.[27] Many of these points are acupuncture points that when stimulated alleviate certain conditions. These conditions are also known to have nutritional remedies; this is how these points were discovered and then correlated with blood tests. In 1981, this author's first discovery in this field, was the finding of this type of nutritional "body (or reflex) point testing" for amino acids. (This wasn't published until 1984.[28]) Finally, we note that we've recently formulated a bio-mathematical model explaining many of the phenomena of Applied Kinesiology or MBT.[29, 30]

Before we begin to perform our first muscle test, we need to list some factors that can affect its accuracy.

PREAMBLE TO MBT (WHEN FEASIBLE)

Look straight ahead during tests
Don't hold breath, can breathe out during actual test
Don't strain or incorporate extraneous muscles or contort during the test. Do your best throughout the test, but if the muscle goes weak, let it go
Remove metal from body, especially electric watches, metal

(jewelry) above the neck or that crosses the body's midline
Don't think negative thoughts which can cause weak responses,
keep the mind "blank"
Wear loose fitting cotton clothes, lighter colors are best
Be in natural lighting
Avoid extraneous sounds
Don't test if subject is hungry or thirsty

Don't worry if you can't test in ideal circumstances. The
preamble below can correct some *"SWITCHING"* that might
be created by less-than-ideal conditions. But be aware that
being switched doesn't just mean your testing may be somewhat
inaccurate. It also means your energy and health are affected.
All these factors can potentially cause what kinesiologists call
"switching" or *NEUROLOGICAL DISORGANIZATION*. I.e.,
they can create imbalances in the body's circuits that can cause
a muscle response opposite to the "unswitched" or true
response. This is similar to connecting wires in a circuit opposite
to the proper way; subsequently a gauge needle may want to
jump the opposite way. There is a temporary unswitching
preamble that can help ensure accuracy. This is crucial as the
E.I. are usually switched! Testing them, without taking these
precautions may be very inaccurate!

UNSWITCHING PREAMBLE FOR SUBJECT AND TESTOR

(1) Rub the navel and the two points above the upper lip and
below the lower lip as in Fig. 8.
(2) Rub the navel and the K27 points. See Fig 8. The K (or
kidney) 27 points are (acupuncture meridian) points under the
collar bone, adjacent to the sternum. (The latter is the bone
running down the center, to which the ribs attach.) Some
kinesiologists say the K27 points must be rubbed daily *until* they
no longer hurt. This relates to neurological disorganization as
described in Ch. 12.

(3) Rub the navel and the coccyx (tailbone) which is just above the anus.

Rub each set of two hand corrections for 5-10 seconds. You can hold the navel (or rub its two "corners" lightly) while more vigorously rubbing the other sets of points. These three corrections temporarily correct top-bottom, left-right, and front-back switching, respectively. These three dimensions are also known as Pitch, Roll and Yaw. (See Ch. 12 for more information on the internal confusion in the body that these relate to.)

Now we're ready. Here we will refer to Figs. 9 and 10. Have the subject extend her arm straight out to the side and stand in front (or back) and off-center a bit. I.e., don't be directly in front. Stabilize the opposite shoulder with your non-testing hand as shown. This helps prevent contortion; some will want to employ muscles other than the one being tested.

MUSCLE TESTING RULES
1. Ask if any injuries are present before start
2. Subject will say "stop" if pain should arise
3. Have several fingers or hand flat on top of the arm just below

Figure 8.

Unswitching Points. Rub these points while holding the navel. Also add the coccyx points (not shown).

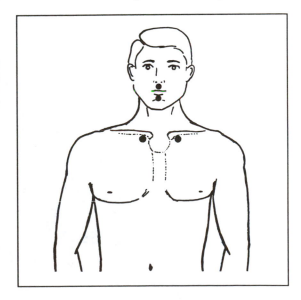

the wrist. Do not grip, or squeeze, the arm

4. Testor will say "hold" just before pressing down towards the floor

5. Testor may show the range of motion to the subject first. I.e., without subject resisting, take the subject's arm and push it down several inches

6. Now the subject will attempt to lock out the muscle and prevent the arm from moving towards the floor as the testor gently begins pushing the arm in this direction

7. Testor builds up pressure *VERY SLOWLY*. During the first second hardly any force is used. This is crucial to allow the subject to actually feel what is occurring!

8. Testor pushes for about 2 seconds

9. With steady pressure, push down the arm only until testor is sure of response. If weak, there's no need to drag the arm down more than 6 inches.

When learning, the most common mistake is to push *too hard, too soon*. A small percentage of people push *too lightly* and don't seem to want to have a weak response show up on their friend. One test for accuracy is to have the subject say a true statement

Figure 9.

Muscle Testing
Procedure.
See also Fig. 10.

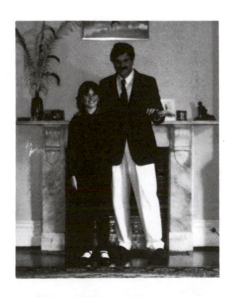

such as his actual name. Quickly muscle test. It should be strong. If the subject says his name is someone else's, he should muscle test weak. This assumes you have taken care of switching.

> **STOP READING NOW! YES, WE MEAN YOU! EITHER TEST SOMEONE RIGHT NOW OR, IF IMPOSSIBLE, CALL SOMEONE RIGHT NOW AND MAKE AN APPOINTMENT FOR MUSCLE TESTING LATER TODAY. THIS IS THE ONLY WAY TO GET WELL RAPIDLY!**

When you're proficient at MBT, you can check for two additional imbalances. Test for dehydration by first testing to see if you have a strong muscle. This is called testing in the clear, as you're not testing anything but the muscle itself. It's also called finding a *"STRONG INDICATOR MUSCLE"* or **SIM**. The dehydration test is to simply (gently) pull some hair on the subject's head while testing the SIM. If the muscle tests weak, provide some pure water and retest in a few seconds. It should now be strong! We're 80% water and dehydration readily weakens (and switches) the body. (Shaky muscles can also result.) Next we will refer to Fig. 11 for testing blood sugar energy imbalance.

Figure 10.

Muscle testing procedure you will start using today!

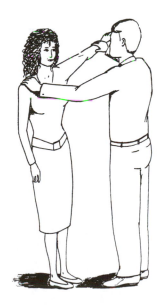

"BLOOD SUGAR ENERGY TEST"

1. Place the thumb one inch above the navel and
2. Simultaneously place the middle and pointer fingers (which are touching each other at the tips) at the point one inch to the subject's left (of the thumb).
3. Test the SIM now.
4. If weak, recommend the subject eat some safe food or perform the energy balance known as the "blood chemistry balance" as described in Ch. 12.

The energy imbalances created by dehydration and faulty blood sugar need to be tested and corrected for accurate MBT.

It will take time to perfect your "feel" or feedback on whether the arm is weak or strong. Vary your pressure with the strength of the subject. Use greater force (but still come in slowly) for the Swartzeneggers and much lesser force for a five year old girl. Remember this is *not* a contest of wills or muscles. It is a test to see if a muscle locks in regard to a specific challenge at the time of the test. The fascinating thing is that a weak response is only 10%, or so, less strong than the "strong" response. This is why this subtle response monitoring wasn't observed until recently by Goodheart.

After some preliminary testing, you should know whether a muscle is strong or not. (This is the whole ball game here.)

Figure 11.

Blood sugar energy test points.

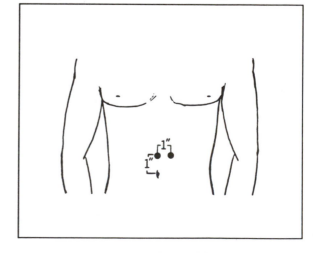

We're now ready to test for environmental sensitivities. The accepted A.K./TFH testing involves chewing a food and keeping it under the tongue for a few seconds. (Preliminary research indicates fair accuracy here.[32] An article in *SCIENCE* proved that a specific signal goes almost immediately from this sublingual region to the brain.[33]) However, we have several objections to this procedure. It can cause a reaction as the substance may enter the blood. It thus can be construed as a "medical" test. Indeed, this is how some clinical ecologists demonstrate allergy, but there MBT is not known or used. There, symptoms are meant to be evoked, and can be medically treated, if need be. It (sublingual MBT) is also not as accurate as the scheme below. Likewise, the accepted kinesiological testing for chemicals is to inhale them. We would put them in vials and test as we do with foods. This way symptoms, as in reactivation of the E-B Virus, are avoided.

Our testing involves "energy" testing only. If a substance (and hence its particular electromagnetic field) is placed on the body (or even up to two inches away), MBT can be utilized with great accuracy! This is hypothesized to work as follows. Every substance has its own characteristic electromagnetic field; and the meridians (near the skin) are also electromagnetic in nature. An allergen would thus have a field that would be disharmonious to the body's meridians (and other) energies.

TESTING FOR SENSITIVITIES[31]

1. Hold the food over each of the first five regions or points.
2. Touch the points for #5 while placing foods at or near the navel. We use the *TESTING SCHEME* shown in Fig. 12.

Region 1 involves the pancreas/spleen. Region 2 is the liver. Point 3 is the "triple warmer alarm point" of Acupuncture theory, an inch below the navel. (This point measures endocrine imbalance.) Region 4 is the thymus. Region 5 is the blood sugar test again. Hold these points while the testing is done to indicate which substances cause this type of imbalance. Regions 6 are the brain hemispheres. All substances should be strong everywhere!

If weak at one place, stop as you have uncovered an energy sensitivity. And never press the substance into the body, rather gently hold against (or even a fraction of an inch away) from the body. Pressing into the body can create pain (which may not even be felt) that can weaken a muscle test.

This scheme is a guide that should be changed if the circumstances warrant it. E.g., if a physician suspects a food is causing arthritis at the knee, he can place the food *there* and test! Most HEBS grads use the *first four* points or regions most of the time. (Over half of a person's sensitivities seem to involve liver or pancreas energy imbalance.) These results may not show up on "medical allergy" testing. Most of these tests are known to be inaccurate for foods. And we are not calling this testing "allergy" anyway. But the MBT testing can pick up *95%* of a person's "sensitivities."

Always test a mono (or single item) food, not combo foods. The question of amount may be an issue. A tiny piece of an

Figure 12.

Testing Scheme.

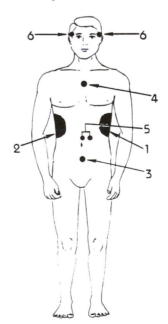

apple may seem O.K., but a whole apple may not. Don't leave foods lying on the body for more than 10 seconds as the body's energies may "adapt" to the stress. Many people buy plastic or glass vials — try the yellow pages for nearby scientific or laboratory supply companies — and collect your own pure foods for testing. Always have an exact control available. Some use prepared kits of homeopathic dilutions. These are in alcohol and will detect only "allergies" and not "sensitivities" which are more prevalent in most individuals.

This fantastic testing offers possibilities that all other testing can't!! You can test fluorescents, T.V.'s, sounds, colors etc. You can test things by looking at them or by being under or near them; as long as your senses pick it up. Getting back to food, if an apple gives a weak response, you can separately test the skin, seeds, and meat. If the skin "is weak," it may be mold or pesticide. Try an organic apple!

We have found that previous and accepted MBT methods for *TESTING SUPPLEMENTS (vitamins)* and very nutritious foods are often inaccurate. This is because sublingual and even body-placement testing can be fooled if the body desperately needs the nutrient. This can cause a strong response even if an allergy is actually present. We are saddened to see some kinesiologists repeatedly tell their patients a supplement is O.K.; and then the patient continually gets sick! *Never* allow yourself to be tested for vitamins except by the following method. *SIMPLY BREAK OFF THE TINIEST PIECE AND USE THE SAME POINTS OF FIG. 12 FOR TESTING!*[34]

We note that skin and blood allergy tests have some limitations superseded by MBT. How do you know what part of the food is in the sample tested? How can you make alterations? But everything has some limitations too. If enzyme or digestive problems exist, MBT may give a false negative. (This may mean its not the food but a digestive failure or even a conditioned response that can be fixed with the "Phobia Cure" of Ch. 15.) We've tested some who said they were allergic to "everything" and it is usually not verified by MBT. Of course, we consider the possibility that HEBS testing is inaccurate, but we believe digestive difficulty (e.g., dumping syndrome) or conditioned response explains the results. Here testing (eating) in an ecological unit would appear to back up the patient, but could still be in error.

We should note that rarely a "reaction" during MBT may occur, even though no substance has been placed *in* the body! We've seen people sneeze when pollen vials are placed on the thymus. And hyperactive children "do their thing" when sugar was placed on the body. But these are exceptions and short-lived. Always remember, the most accurate test is reality itself. But MBT, when used optimally, can be the quickest, least expensive, least "symptom-provoking" and most accurate test available! But be aware that we are testing for energy imbalance and not "medical" allergy.

Figs. 13 and 14 depict the recent development of *"SELF-TESTING."* You can test yourself for any imbalance in this book in this way! Self-testing may never be as accurate as having an "external" testor. But this may not be available. After unswitching yourself, use your fingers as shown. Press the middle finger onto the pointer finger. (Resist the pressure, of course.) Some use the ring finger as the "muscle" to be tested because it can "give" more readily. Check for accuracy by saying "yes" and "no" separately as you test yourself. The first should be strong, the second, weak.

Finally, we describe a method which will enable you to test a small child or anyone whose muscles are too feeble (or too strong) to be tested directly!

SURROGATE TESTING

1. Test the surrogate's arm, with no contact with the subject, to make sure you have a strong indicator muscle. See Fig. 15.
2. Test the surrogate while she holds hands with the actual subject. (Some other skin contact could also be used.) This

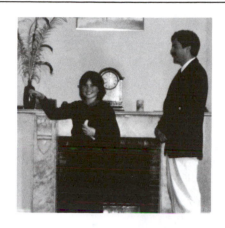
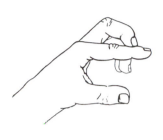

Figure 13 & Figure 14.

Self-testing.

should test strong. If not, some imbalance, e.g. emotional, occurs when the contact is made.

3. Now place the food on the subject (or touch the various testing points [on the subject] of the next three chapters) and test the *surrogate's* arm.

If it goes weak, it is a sensitivity on the part of the subject and *not* the surrogate because the food is on the subject! There is nothing "mystical" about this (or anything else in MBT). It is analogous to something demonstrated in biofeedback. We've seen the following set-up. The subject is touching a surrogate. The latter is hooked up to an electrical device which sounds an alarm when stress is detected. But an alarm is sounded when the surrogate is calm and the *subject* thinks of a stressful situation. The energy is passed along to the surrogate just as in MBT. In MBT, the need for expensive electrical devices is obviated!

Figure 15.

Surrogate Testing.

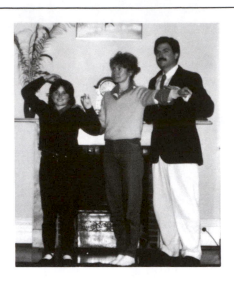

10

BRAIN HEMISPHERE INTEGRATION: THE DYSLEXIA CONNECTION

We're ready to use our new MBT skills as we enter the fascinating realm of brain hemispheric integration. We will see that the ecologically ill and the dyslexic have much in common. Yes, the spaceyness, poor memory and coordination in the E.I., and the inability to read in the dyslexic, have the same lack of brain integration as the cause in many cases. Though the person stricken with E.I. may not want to realize *he* is dyslexic, and the dyslexic (or his parents) may not want to realize *he* is ecologically ill — these two maladies are deeply intertwined! And you can be very intelligent and have a lack of brain integration. Indeed many with E.I. and dyslexia are highly intelligent. The E.I. may no longer be able to manifest it and the dyslexic may never have had the opportunity! After examining the simple theory behind this discovery, we'll go over simple exercises that can correct many of these imbalances!

Let's start by taking a look at dyslexia. Literally it means an inability to read. In reality, it is a continuum of reading difficulty with *80%* of Americans experiencing occasional "mild" forms of reading difficulty! The "experts" have variously viewed dyslexia as caused by emotional problems, eye or ear disorders and drug deficiencies. The last may involve treatment with antihistamines. This may be a warped and roundabout way of linking dyslexia to allergies. A book by clinical ecologist, Doris Rapp,

M.D., depicts the handwritings of dyslexics (showing transposed letters) along with normal writing after treatment with neutralization injections for allergens.[35]

Going beyond allergies, this author has linked dyslexia to the effects of two chemicals. These are formaldehyde and acetaldehyde. Both belong to a class of chemicals called aldehydes. How can these substances cause reading problems? To answer this, we need to look at the two brain hemispheres.

Much information on the differences between the left and right halves of the brain has been gained in the last 100 years. Research has been gathered from experiments on people with brain injuries or from those who have had surgical separation of their brain hemispheres. The left hemisphere is more analytical and temporal; it's in charge of logic, language and mathematical abilities. The right half is more emotional, musical, spatial and global. It supposedly sees the "whole picture" and is therefore called the "gestalt" hemisphere. (In some people the usual functions of the two hemispheres are transposed; but this is rare, despite the claims of some kinesiologists.)

The two brain hemispheres are joined by the tissue, or set of nerve fibers, known as the *CORPUS CALLOSUM* (and by some smaller, less important structures called commisures.) It is the corpus callosum, we assert that is not functioning properly in dyslexics and most of the E.I. Though the E.I. may not have "total dyslexia," they will report frequent episodes of falling asleep or tiring while reading, or having to reread lines. (Many will admit to not reading much. Some may even claim any book they read is too complicated, because they are not yet aware of this problem or too afraid to do something about it. Don't let this happen to you! Read on and do the simple correction in this chapter.) Their poor memory, often for names, is definitely linked to brain integration problems. (We may leave out the "hemisphere" in "brain hemisphere integration," henceforth.)

Other signs of this type of problem that we see in the ecologically ill include the following. Many when asked to touch the left eye will touch the right or waver indecisively for many seconds. Their personal letters to me often contain transposed letters. Sometimes an "8" is written discontinuously as two little "o's" one on top of the other. This probably indicates other related imbalances in Pitch, Roll and Yaw found in Ch. 12. What the faulty eight reveals is that the adult had a brain imbalance as a child—while learning to write. Taken with difficulty in riding a merry-go-round or car sickness, these learning problems correlate with the term we have coined, *"PRE-CAN-DIDIASIS IMBALANCE."* These learning and spinning problems show up long before serious, more (well-known) physical problems do.

Now what happens as we read? We read from left to right and when the eyes are left-most in their sockets (the left field of vision), the opposite (i.e., the right) brain hemisphere is primarily "activated." Similarly, when looking at the right visual field, the left brain is activated. This is an example of the cross lateralness of all birds and mammals. You know that the left brain (hemisphere) controls the right side of the body and vice versa. If a person suffers a stroke in the left hemisphere, it is the *right* side of the body that may be paralyzed. Now the stress of reading, if any, occurs as the eyes move from the left field (right brain activated) towards the midline. Before proper control can be transferred to the left brain (for viewing the right visual field), the midline is crossed. This activates the corpus callosum. If it is not functioning properly, problems will then occur. Anything from having to reread the line to a total inability to read can result. Transposing letters, like "b" for "d" or seeing and writing a backwards "e" are also possible.

The link to remembering names (in the E.I.) is clearly a similar type of problem. Research on those who have had lobotomies or surgical separation of the hemispheres shows that many can see and "know" what an object is when viewed off to one side, or held by the hand on that side, but cannot possibly *say* its name! The two hemispheres just can't communicate with each other! The different manifestations of reading and other cerebral problems is due to the continuum of corpus callosum dysfunction. (Note that Orientals, who read vertically, may be spared the stress of horizontal reading.)

Now let's look at some treatments offered for dyslexics. The "experts" say 10-20% of American children have dyslexic problems. "Special education" classes and teachers have become commonplace and entail their own bureaucracy. Dyslexics often spend thousands of dollars on visual devices, psychiatric "help" or go "underground" in their adult life utilizing tape recorders or tutors, friends and spouses to help out. Many are left back in school or progress very slowly. We assert that emotional stress surely results, but is never a cause!

Now let's look at a fascinating, but simple type of exercise called cross-crawl. Cross-crawling involves simultaneously using the left and right sides of the body. Walking and running properly are cross-crawls. Some aerobic exercises and proper ski technique are also cross-crawls. (See how many have trouble doing them.) Drs. Doman and Delacato of Pennsylvania were the first to use cross-crawling for those with learning problems or neurological disorders, over 30 years ago. They had people lift up the right arm and left leg simultaneously and then drop them down and pick up the left arm and right leg. You can try this now. Cross-crawling was incorporated into A.K. by Goodheart and into TFH by Thie. Numerous other kinesiologists made refinements in the last 10 years. Some had dyslexics first perform "homolateral crawl" (a same-side arm and leg raising exercise) for months if they could not cross-crawl. The rationale is that "normal" infants first crawl homolaterally, switching over to cross-crawl after a year or so. Some kinesiologists said that dyslexia resulted from "crawling the wrong way at the wrong time." As a physicist, this strikes me as too metaphorical. Because the question immediately arises, *why* didn't (or couldn't) the infant crawl properly at the appropriate time? By 1983, several kinesiologists had come up with ways of correcting dyslexia. Some used variations of cross-crawl and some (chiropractic physicians) employed cranial manipulations. This author entered this field in 1983 and attempted to unify ecology, kinesiology and learning theory.

A basic piece of the puzzle came from Truss in 1984. He asserted that much of the harm done by Candida resulted from its waste product, acetaldehyde. This chemical can affect the metabolic, neurological, endocrine and immune systems. Truss indicated that few chemicals could create so much havoc in the body, as acetaldehyde can. It may interfere with the receptors for acetylcholine — supposedly the major neurotransmitter in the corpus callosum. This researcher then immediately performed some kinesiological experiments. While waiting for acetaldehyde to arrive from a chemical supply company, the experiment below was performed with dilutions of formaldehyde. The latter is the next (and smallest) "brother" of acetaldehyde in the aldehyde chain of chemicals. Now, by this time there were simple exercises to correct dyslexia in minutes, or even seconds. (Yes, you read right.) We performed these cross-crawl corrections with dilutions of formaldehyde taped to dyslexics right brain hemispheres. Result: the expected brain hemispheric integration or repatterning did not occur! Next we performed advanced, priority, energy balancing for Candida or formaldehyde. This led to brain integration intrinsically without the need to repattern with exercises. When the acetaldehyde arrived, I duplicated the results done with formaldehyde. Similar results with other toxic chemicals were not observed.

By Dec. 1984, I had formulated the **ROCHLITZ ALDEHYDE DYSLEXIA HYPOTHESIS**[36,37] or **RADH**. The RADH states that either (or both) of these aldehydes can adversely affect the corpus callosum. In particular, the connection of this tissue to the right brain hemisphere (or less frequently the left) is interfered with. (A year after formulating this hypothesis we received a paper that noted that biochemist Steven Barker, Ph.D., wrote in a 1980 issue of the *JOURNAL OF MEDICAL*

HYPOTHESES that formaldehyde may be the cause of schizophrenia[38] – another brain integration disorder!) Kinesiologists use the term "switched off," as do some neurobiologists. Thus the corpus callosum, and especially its connection to the right brain hemisphere, is switched off in dyslexics by an aldehyde. Some kinesiologists and many others in the health movement say the right brain is switched off. But we think it is the connection of it to the corpus callosum that is at fault. Recent reports appear to back this up; dyslexics are said to have excellent peripheral vision. And the right brain is "on" when viewing the left visual field; only when approaching the midline does a problem arise. While activating the right brain is "in" these days, it bears reminding how many have some aversion to science and logic nowadays. These wonderful functions have left brain involvement. Of course, the ability to have both hemispheres simultaneously activated is the key here.

As the liver detoxifies aldehydes, in some cases, it may be "switched off" too. A corollary of the RADH states that to correct dyslexia with a repatterning exercise, whatever systems are switched off need to be "simultaneously" innervated or switched on. We will demonstrate this graphically below.

Let's first look at the aldehydes in more detail. *FORMAL-DEHYDE* is now fairly well known. It is a ubiquitous environmental toxin. It's toxic, allergenic and carcinogenic and is found in building and insulating materials, wood products, clothing, foam (hypoallergenic??) pillows, rugs, cosmetics (now banned in the U.S.) and even in water and milk. If you have a "100%" cotton shirt that is "sanforized" or "permanent pressed," it's been treated with formaldehyde. Formaldehyde is also produced from Aspartame. Though sold under different brand names, it is the major artificial sweetener, around the world, at this time.

Aspartame contains the amino acids aspartic acid and phenylalanine and also 10% methanol. This is the "rot-gut" alcohol that killed or blinded people when the usual alcohol (ethanol) was banned during the American Prohibition of the 20's. It is the methanol that is processed into formaldehyde in the body. Very recent research indicates that many people are susceptible to neurological and other symptoms from ingesting Aspartame. [C,D,E,F]

Formaldehyde is also produced in the body. It is a metabolic waste product (as in amino acid metabolism) and is hopefully short-lived. Formaldehyde is among the worst offenders for the E.I. It also became infamous after the Arab oil embargo of 1973. A foam derivative was used as an insulation in many homes. Everything from headaches to phlebitis resulted! (We will see that loss of brain and heart integration are among the first symptoms!) Formaldehyde is also used to preserve cadavers. Several physicians have told us that allergies and health problems began during their first year in medical school when they worked extensively with cadavers. (Some have even noted that this may be when some physicians-to-be lose their capacity to see the whole picture, as brain integration may have been lost.) The liver has enzymes to detoxify it. These enzymes are limited in amount and also must detoxify acetaldehyde, if present.

Acetaldehyde has several known sources. It is a fungal (and not bacterial) waste product. It is also found in cigarette smoke (as is formaldehyde), smog (including auto exhaust) and alcoholic beverages. Unlike formaldehyde, acetaldehyde is not an internal metabolic product. It is supposedly far more harmful to the body than is formaldehyde. Now if the mother has some (possibly unknown) Candida problem, we assert that the fetus may be born with a propensity towards dyslexia or hyperactivity. The Candida problem may be vaginal or uterine, but *need not be* as acetaldehyde is very volatile and can enter the blood and travel anywhere. Thus intestinal Candida overgrowth could be the cause. The acetaldehyde could "switch off" brain integration before the baby-to-be ever gets a chance. As we have said, "it's no coincidence that the epidemic of dyslexia and hyperactivity in children is occurring simultaneous with the epidemic of vaginal and other Candida problems in the mothers of these children!" This is why the baby "crawls the wrong way at the wrong time." If the baby is otherwise genetically strong, no other manifestation of illness may result.

Here in this new edition of *ALLERGIES AND CANDIDA: WITH THE PHYSICIST'S RAPID SOLUTION*, we want you to know that one of our predictions has been verified. An article in *SCIENCE*[G,H] has found that acetaldehyde does cross the placental barrier and causes fetal brain damage. The study was about acetaldehyde from alcoholic beverages, but clearly this applies to acetaldehyde in the mother's body which has been produced by Candida overgrowth. (We first reported this in our newsletter.)

Thus brain integration is among the most fragile of energy systems in the body (and thus the hardest to maintain). This is why some super-healthy athletes are known to be dyslexic. Olympic decathlon champion Bruce Jenner and the greatest diver who ever lived, Olympic champion, Greg Luganis are examples. Both are unlikely to have any Candida overgrowth! Once again we see that the conceptualization of clinical ecology (at present) is somewhat limiting. Both are known to be dyslexic. Jenner has to study for hours before doing a broadcast, often with friends or his spouse. With Luganis we note an interesting, possible Candida tie-in. Written reports have him saying that he often drank a case of beer during lunch breaks in high school. Thus while lack of brain integration may be the only imbalance in these remarkable athletes, most other dyslexic children have many other problems. Many are known to have asthma, hay fever and more systemic forms of allergy.

Prof. Geschwind of Harvard had his own unique theories about dyslexia.[39] He performed autopsies on numerous dyslexics. He frequently found the left hemisphere was larger than the right, especially in males. (He noted that many dyslexics have significant mathematical abilities.) Prof. Geschwind theorized that fetal chemical abnormalities with the sex hormone, testosterone, led to underdevelopment of the right (and overdevelopment of the left) hemisphere. With the RADH, we would assert that this is another result not a cause. Indeed, Truss outlined that acetaldehyde affects the sex hormones, including testosterone. The RADH may be the first consistent and "complete" theory of dyslexia. We only hope that some physicians will undertake a study of levels of the two aldehydes in dyslexics, before and after our repatterning exercises and other corrections.

Now we're ready to leave the theory and go to a simple "hands on" testing for the lack of brain integration.

TESTING FOR BRAIN HEMISPHERE INTEGRATION

1. Perform the same muscle test as before and make sure it is strong in the clear. (Finding a S.I.M., you recall.)
2. Now draw a large "X" on a blank piece of paper
3. Hold it directly (about 10 inches) in front of the subject at their eye level
4. Simultaneously, muscle test again—this is the actual test

If weak, you have uncovered a lack of brain integration. Don't diagnose dyslexia, because that's just a name and you will momentarily make the correction anyway.

We include a perhaps frightening aside here. With this subtle type of testing, a large percentage of the population—especially the young—are being found to have "dyslexic tendency". This relates to many problems or idiosyncrasies in society today. Including the younger generation's problems with alcohol, drugs, crime, and even the toxic music prevalent. Let's examine the last factor. Some would say music is aesthetic and we can't judge it this way. But again, MBT of the rock beat will test weak on everyone. Now the rock beat is a musical variation that could theoretically have taken place anytime in the last 500 years or more. Why now? It began in the 1950's just when antibiotics were getting "big". What we are saying is that Candida or acetaldehyde caused dyslexic patterning. Only dyslexic brains would devise such music and only a dyslexic generation (or portion thereof) would become addicted to it. Sure enough, as the 60's and 70's came and went, rock music became more warped. Hard rock, heavy metal and rap music are "in". Rap music is an almost undisguised, discontinuous or dyslexic-like talking. It is fascinating that the most ecologically ill — unable to tolerate, or become addicted to, drugs or smoking or coffee — have a history of also being unable to tolerate rock music. This author sometimes felt left out in his youth because he intrinsically felt weakened or sickened by much of his generation's music. But this would also be true of most scientists.

Let's go beyond testing for dyslexia and see how quickly we can overcome it. The correction is the simple brain integration exercise.

HEBS BRAIN INTEGRATION EXERCISE

1. Do a cross-crawl by touching the right hand over to the left knee (as the knee is raised up from the floor) while humming. Keep the arm straight (at the elbow) throughout. See Fig. 16.
2. Drop the hand and leg as soon as they touch and then
3. Do the same thing with the left hand and right leg.
4. Repeat this for a minute or two.
5. You will sequentially use each pair of opposite arm and leg during this exercise. Do steps 1-5 for a while first before adding #6.
6. The final step is to slowly, visually track (look at) all the points along a large circle in front of you, as you continue the exercise. First gaze along a clockwise direction and then counterclockwise.

You may want to use a mirror or have someone watch you, if you are spacey. Wanting to touch the same side arm and leg may be a sign of "dyslexic tendency." This is a desire to perform homolateral crawl as cross-crawl is not yet "switched on."

You can do everything slowly, if you like. Your partner may

"trace" the circle with a hand, or pen, while standing in front of you. Keep the head facing straight in front, use only your eyes for the tracking. This visual tracking makes use of the fact that different regions of the brain are activated while the eyes look in different, corresponding regions.[40] When you're done, re-test looking at the "X."

Some people may need to do this correction while counting (the left, not the right, hemisphere would be switched off here) instead of humming. Your test result will indicate this; i.e., if the "X" still tests weak, perform the whole procedure while *counting*. This would then be step #7. It should now be strong.

> **STOP READING NOW! YES, WE MEAN YOU! DO THIS SIMPLE CORRECTION NOW! DO IT, IF YOU WANT TO BE WELL. THERE ARE NO MAGIC PILLS THAT WILL GET YOU WELL! DON'T READ THIS BOOK LIKE A HISTORY BOOK—IT'S A SELF-HELP MANUAL. YES, YOU CAN DO THE CORRECTION EVEN WITHOUT TESTING IT. IT CAN'T HURT YOU! THE PHYSICIST'S RAPID SOLUTION WILL HAVE YOU FEELING BETTER ALMOST IMMEDIATELY AFTER YOU TAKE THESE FIRST STEPS.**

Figure 16.
H.E.B.S. Brain Integration Exercise. Add the Hum (or count) then the visual tracking while performing it. Touch the opposite side of the opposite knee; use both pairs of opposite arm-and-leg. Like walking!!

Left figure: One half—the right arm and left leg combination. Right figure: The left arm and right leg combination.

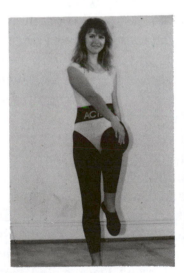
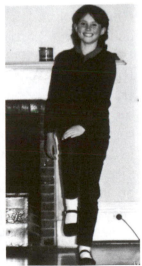

You may want to have the subject read aloud—before and after—the correction. You may want to tape this as many with E.I., and dyslexia, can be close-minded to rapid corrections! This exercise can help alleviate "classical dyslexia" as well!

How does it work? The author was the first to explain this. Let's return to the RADH. To correct dyslexic patterning, we said that we needed to simultaneously activate the right brain, corpus callosum and possibly the liver. This exercise does precisely this. Any cross-crawl activates the corpus callosum. (This is why cross-crawl is difficult for the dyslexic, and the E.I.) Humming activates especially the right brain hemisphere. And the particular hand motion (touching the opposite knee) utilizes the A.K./TFH muscles for the brain (mostly) and liver. Recall that A.K./TFH realizes a specific muscle/meridian/organ connection. This arm motion involves muscles that are connected to the brain (primarily) and the liver. (These muscles are the supraspinatus and the rhomboids, but this doesn't matter here.)

Dyslexic cross-crawl corrections were realized since about 1982, but this author was the first to explain how they work in 1985. Another brain integration exercise is the HEBS "Chicken Crawl" pictured in Fig. 17. Always do both pairs of opposite arm and leg. Don't forget the hum and visual tracking of the circle. If visual tracking makes you dizzy, *STOP* and skip to the Pitch, Roll and Yaw corrections of Ch. 12. Once switched on, cross-crawling is very beneficial. The hum and tracking can be left out, if you remain switched on. (Just test the "X", if you're not sure.) This correction is not "permanent," as E.I. (and perhaps) aldehyde build-up can recur. Unfortunately, some kinesiologists claim permanent cures or corrections. Clearly, in an age of chocolate and Chernobyls, this is nonsense!

The two most popular kinesiologies that dealt with brain integration also said that homolateral crawl should test weak for optimum functioning. This is in error. (Those who tested strong on homolateral crawl were called "dumb athletes.")

Indeed, schizophrenics are said to have enlarged corpus cal-losums.[41] They may be *too* integrated. Perhaps they can't keep some strange thoughts in only one brain hemisphere as the rest of us can! One should be strong for all types of physical ac-tivity![42] An additional advanced concept is the author's dis-covery of *META-INTEGRATION*. This is the first consistent explanation of how the brain contains both homolateral and cross-lateral components (thoughts or movement feedback) in it at *all* times. Even the eyes have connections to both brain hemispheres. And when doing a homolateral crawl, the brain's hemispheres control the opposite side of the body. Thus cross-lateral and homolateral components can never be truly isolated. They are approximations. Meta-integration coincides with known holographic properties of the brain.[43]

Advanced HEBS Brain Integration schemes can even be employed for those who are crippled and can't crawl. They involve looking at the "X" and humming and strengthening certain muscles simultaneously. This can be used instead of, (or better) in addition to, the very expensive cross-crawl machines that have helped those with neurological and neuromuscular disorders.

Brain integration exercises are very beneficial for the E.I. They can be performed twice a day. You may feel clearer and more energetic, coordinated and balanced. Of course, you will likely read more and remember better. This is just the beginning! It's just the first step in our discussion of what kinesiologists call neurological disorganization.

Now even though integrated in the general sense, specific emotional issues may test weak when thought of and while viewing an "X." Here nutrition is the key. The anti-aldehyde nutrients listed in Ch. 7 may be very beneficial. Molybdenum, we believe is the major anti-aldehyde nutrient. When Molyb-denum is placed under the tongue, the issue may be de-stressed, if thought of at the same time!

Finally we note that the corpus callosum, like all brain cells have a high metabolic rate. They therefore need much oxygen and glucose. Undoubtedly, hypoglycemia and low oxygen states (as are found in the E.I.) can cause the corpus callosum to malfunction; even though no aldehyde imbalance is involved. Recently, pesticides, organic solvents and even food components have been found to affect learning and memory; and formaldehyde was found to be one of these. (See Ref. 72.) This, recall, was ascertained by the author, only with MBT! (To help avoid learning and other neurological problems, don't have infants crawl on new rugs, which emit both formaldehyde and pesticides.) The same chemicals are being linked to Alzheimer's Disease, Parkinson's and other degenerative brain disorders.

Figure 17.

The H.E.B.S. Chicken Crawl.

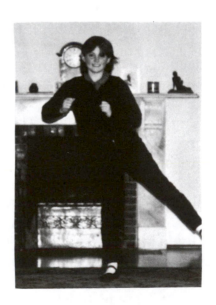

11

HEART INTEGRATION™: THE "DYSLEXIC HEART" CONNECTION

In 1985, this author discovered a kinesiological correction that may have wide importance in ecology, cardiology and learning theory. Another set of common complaints in the E.I. are cold hands and feet, pale complexion, faulty blood pressure (usually low), cardiac arrhythmias, stiffness and achiness. (Recall the Coca pulse test which shows that the heart rate changes from allergic reactions.) Likewise, many dyslexics and allergic children have pale faces and even the cold hands and feet. I can recall these complaints as a young child. These complaints in the E.I. are often not alleviated by any treatment, analogous to the "brain complaints" of the last chapter. Some physicians routinely treat the cold hands and feet with thyroid medication. (Sometimes, appropriate testing isn't done.)

Let's look at some theory first. The heart has hemispheres with slightly differing functions, somewhat analogous to the brain. The beating of the heart's four chambers and the peripheral pulses often are not at the same frequency. The Soviets consider the heart to be a "second brain" with holographic qualities. Western researchers have recently discovered that the heart is an endocrine gland,[44] producing hormones that regulate blood pressure and interact with the other organs including the kidneys and the brain. It is far more than a simple pump. (This chapter may indicate why mechanical hearts may never work!) We all know that allegory has it that thoughts and feelings are "in the heart."

This author discovered, in 1985, that the heart hemispheres can become "dyslexic" too. We use this term because it depicts a heart not functioning in an integrated manner—a heart out of "synch" with itself and the brain. Another RADH corollary is that aldehydes (or other substances) may lead to dyslexic heart. This condition may not show up on an EKG as dyslexia does not show up on EEG's. (Recent computerized interpretations of EEG's do *at last* reveal a dyslexic profile.[45] Perhaps one day my discovery of dyslexic heart will also be observed.)

We will reveal two simple exercises to correct dyslexic heart. But first, let's see how to test for it.

HEART INTEGRATION™ TESTING SCHEME

1. Use the deltoid, or some other SIM, and place the subject's hand over his heart. This should test strong.
2. Next, with the hand still over the heart, hold up the "X".
3. If the muscle is weak on viewing the "X", dyslexic heart exists.
[Note: Heart Integration™ is a registered trademark of Prof. Steven Rochlitz.]

This is not a medical condition! Someone with a heart disease may well test strong, signaling an integrated heart. And someone with a perfect heart may test weak—the hemispheres, at the moment, are not integrated.

Now let's look at our first correction. This 1985 discovery was devised to correct the author's arrhythmia which occurred as an allergic reaction. (It did that immediately.)

ROCHLITZ HEART INTEGRATION™ EXERCISE[46]

1. It is another cross-crawl variant; use opposite arm and leg again. Start out with the right arm as shown in Fig. 18.
2. As best as you comfortably can, hold the elbow up at shoulder

height and out to the side with the lower arm (and hand) making a right angle with the upper arm. I.e., the hand and forearm are pointing down at the floor. This is the scarecrow starting position.
3. Next rotate at the shoulder (arm and hand as they were). That is, keep the scarecrow, just rotate at the shoulder towards the left side.
4. As the elbow reaches the midline, flick up the forearm towards the horizontal. Now the following is not depicted in the photos; but instead of stopping the forearm at the horizontal position (as is shown), you can continue to rotate the forearm (at the elbow) until the hand is pointing up to the sky. This is the optimum exercise.
5. *At this exact time*, bring up the opposite (left) knee.
6. Then let them both drop down. I.e., the arm drops back to the side while the leg drops to the floor.
7. Repeat with the other pair of opposite arm and leg. Be careful *not* to do this in a homolateral (same side arm and leg) way.
8. Do this while humming. Note the brain-heart communication which has been verified biochemically.[47] (A few will need to count to "switch it on.")
9. Add the visual circular tracking as in the brain integration exercise.

This exercise apparently can integrate the brain as well as the heart. Some call it the Rochlitz Scarecrow Exercise. We refer to Figs. 18 through Fig. 21. If you lose your balance, it is not because the exercise is terribly difficult, rather you may have poor balance. This is usually due to other circuits malfunctioning; especially brain integration or *Pitch, Roll and Yaw*. (See the next Chapter.) You can skip to them now if you need to. Don't give up! As with all the corrections in this book, if you find them difficult to do or understand, get a friend or relative to help you out!! Do the exercise for a minute or two. If you are forbidden to exercise, perhaps the next correction below may be less strenuous. If you are huffing because you don't exercise, maybe it's time to start! This exercise as well as the brain integration exercise can be done while lying in bed.
    When you've finished, retest heart integration as you first did.

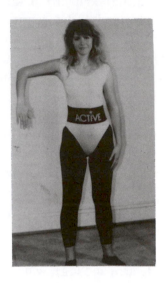
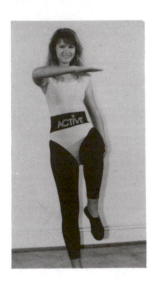
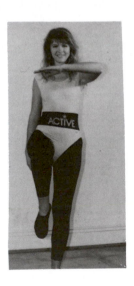
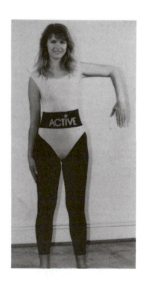

Figure 18 - Figure 21.

Rochlitz Heart Integration Exercise. Going clockwise, from the top left: First half starting position, the first half completed, second half starting position, the second half completed.

It should now test strong. (If weak, do it again while counting.)

STOP READING NOW! YES, WE MEAN YOU! DO THIS SIMPLE CORRECTION NOW! DO IT, IF YOU WANT TO BE WELL. THERE ARE NO MAGIC PILLS THAT WILL GET YOU WELL! DON'T READ THIS BOOK LIKE A HISTORY BOOK – IT'S A SELF-HELP MANUAL. YES, YOU CAN DO THE CORRECTION EVEN WITHOUT TESTING IT. IT CAN'T HURT YOU! THE PHYSICIST'S RAPID SOLUTION WILL HAVE YOU FEELING BETTER ALMOST IMMEDIATELY AFTER YOU TAKE THESE FIRST STEPS.

You may feel stronger, more energetic and even less foggy. This exercise is perhaps the most important correction for those with M.S. (Multiple Sclerosis), especially if *one side* is worse than the other. It apparently gets both blood and nerve "energy" flowing. We saw one woman with a bad M.S. limp and a loss of sensation in one foot, for 15 years, get sensation back in the foot in *seconds*. She then ran! Her ankle also unswelled before us in seconds! HEBS Grad, Ann McAlpin Cain, reports that it prevented serious injury after her horse knocked her down. Her mother also prevented bruising after bashing her shin. We've seen it unfreeze frozen muscles too. An Australian student reported great immediate improvement in his varicose veins.

It helps to have "hard evidence" and we do have it. First we've seen it normalize, or at least lower, high blood pressure in minutes. We have the printouts as proof. Unfortunately, they don't copy well. We do hand them out at the seminars. It can normalize (raise) low blood pressure, but this is harder to see right away. This is because any exercise tends to raise blood pressure. This makes the lowering of high blood pressure all the more remarkable.

Another visual "proof" is the following. We make use of changes in leg abduction (or spreading apart). With your friend lying on a table or the floor, mark (below, on the floor) the exact spot that they can abduct (spread) a leg out to the side, stopping at the point when pain begins. Mark the big toe's position. Also mark where their head and hips were. You want to make sure you put them back in the same starting position. If the person is on a table, mark the spot vertically below their toe. Use the leg that has more circulatory difficulty for this procedure. If heart integration is achieved, retest. We've seen changes of six inches to three feet! (Changes of less than three inches are insignificant.) Even those with "great stretches" show marked improvement. One dancer was finally able to wrap her leg around her neck. How could this happen? Answer: If the adductor muscle in the leg stretches much better, it can only mean it has a better supply of blood. But this must be true of the entire body!! Many feel their hands warming up within seconds or minutes. (But dietary concerns, we shall see, can override this correction.)

A variation of this exercise may be known in the Soviet Union! Most troops march in cross-crawl fashion, with the swinging arm either coming straight up or going towards the opposite knee. On May Day, you can see the Soviets march with the arm making a similar flick up to the opposite side. (Of course the gun prevents utilizing the opposite pair of limbs. And they don't start out with the optimum scarecrow position.)

We are the first to explicitly relate this type of arm motion to the heart, but we've also seen other indications that some athletes intrinsically know something about this. Tap dancers have a routine that uses the arms like our Maestro (see the next page) while their legs also move out to the side. Likewise, jumping rope — one of the best and most exacting of aerobic exercises — also appears to be a variation of the HEBS Maestro exercise. You can also rent the video of the movie, *THE MUSIC MAN*, and watch Robert Preston march along while flicking his opposite arm very much like our heart integration exercise! So maybe we got there (intrinsically speaking) before the Soviets.

Our exercise may indeed be the best for improving circulation!! Athletes report great energy boosts even if they've always had heart integration. It apparently increases heart output.

Our second heart integration exercise is called the *HEBS MAESTRO*. We became aware that some studies showed that exercising with the arms may be *better* (cardiovascularly) than the usual running or walking exercises. This "arm jogging" is clearly performed by music conductors, many of whom live to their nineties.[48] A medical kinesiologist claimed the conductor has more "life energy" or "thymus energy." That may be, but again sounds too metaphorical. After Fred Shull, M.D. sent us an article on arm jogging, we pondered this issue and immediately had the answer. The music conductor is performing a heart integration exercise! He is using both arms, is humming or carrying a tune, and is looking all around him! Just as with the Rochlitz Heart Integration, this exercise integrates and strengthens the heart. Both exercises are great cardiovascular exercises. Repeated use apparently continues to keep the heart at an optimum. We have had reports of the HEBS Maestro being performed on National TV (and in the national press) by the 1400 pound man, Walter Hudson!

Here's how to do the second heart integration exercise. See Fig. 22.

HEBS MAESTRO

1. With the elbows high and out to the side a bit, trace (with your hands, not your eyes) two "C's" that are back to back.
2. Add the hum and the circular, visual tracking.

STOP READING NOW! YES, WE MEAN YOU! DO THIS SIMPLE CORRECTION NOW! DO IT, IF YOU WANT TO BE WELL. THERE ARE NO MAGIC PILLS THAT WILL GET YOU WELL! DON'T READ THIS BOOK LIKE A HISTORY BOOK – IT'S A SELF-HELP MANUAL. YES, YOU CAN DO THE CORRECTION EVEN WITHOUT TESTING IT. IT CAN'T HURT YOU! THE PHYSICIST'S RAPID SOLUTION WILL HAVE YOU FEELING BETTER ALMOST IMMEDIATELY AFTER YOU TAKE THESE FIRST STEPS.

If pain or stiffness prevents performance of the exact recommen-dations for either heart integration, just do the best you can. It'll be just fine. This exercise, unlike the previous one integrates the heart only and not the brain. You can do the leg abduction test, before and after, here too. This exercise is easier to do, but we believe the first one may be even more beneficial.

How do these two exercises integrate the heart? They were hypothesized by the author as part of the Rochlitz Meridian Integra-tion Theory. Using the A.K./TFH muscle in a cross-crawl (with the hum or count) integrates and strengthens the related organ! Here the subscapularis/heart muscle is used. As with the brain integration exercises, there are no permanent cures in this world. This repat-terning exercise was hypothesized. Since the resulting changes in blood pressure and muscle stretching were predicted, we have the beginnings of a science here.

Though we've seen high blood pressure normalize from these exercises, the dietary factors causing high blood pressure *are* known! The medical profession is lying when they say the cause

Figure 22.

HEBS Maestro.

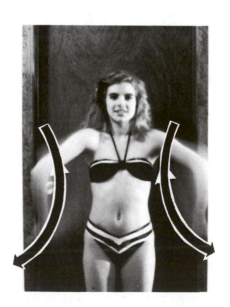

is unknown! Assuming no cardiovascular or kidney disease, most people could normalize their blood pressure on their own! In graduate school, this author came across some nutrition texts written over thirty years ago. They said that many headaches may be due to foods containing a class of chemicals called monoamines. They are vasoactive — they affect the diameter of blood vessels. (We believe any allergy can do this.) Monoamines are found in cheese, wine, anything fermented, coffee, chocolate, citrus, beans, and bananas. I reported this to people even when I was a physicist and always saw people normalize their own blood pressure within days of changing their diet! Assuming, again, no pathology exists; we say that cheese causes high blood pressure most frequently and the most moldy cheese causes the most elevated blood pressure! Salt and cholesterol in the diet are not the cause of high blood pressure. This is another medical myth! If, however, the underlying allergic, nutritional and energy factors in this chapter are not dealt with, salt and cholesterol may worsen the condition.

The circulatory system also needs nutrients to function properly.

CARDIOVASCULAR NUTRIENTS

VITAMINS: C, P (bioflavonoids), E, B_6, lecithin, fish oil-EPA, MINERALS: magnesium, potassium, selenium and silicon AMINO ACIDS: carnitine and taurine; OTHER NUTRIENTS: Coenzyme Q_{10} and mucopolysaccharides. The latter includes carageenan (from seaweed) or CSA from beef aorta tissue.

So while the Rochlitz Heart Integration or HEBS Maestro exercises may normalize blood pressure, if faulty diet is the cause, the correction may not last. This is another example of how the *PHYSICIST'S RAPID SOLUTION* is energy and ecology balancing!

Let's return to the young dyslexic. If he is otherwise perfectly healthy, like a Bruce Jenner or Greg Luganis, heart integration

is undoubtedly maintained. There exists an intrinsic, homeos-
tatic hierarchy in the body. The body, under stress would lose
the less survival-oriented mechanisms *first*. Apparently heart
integration is more crucial than brain integration. The pale,
sickly dyslexic or the allergic child—both are often the same,
we assert—probably has lost heart integration.You will usually
find most who don't have heart integration will also not have
brain integration and not vice versa. The exception appears to
be in the elderly. We have found some senior citizens maintaining brain, but not heart, integration. Again heart integration is
perhaps the most crucial energy imbalance to restore for those
with M.S. Brain integration and Pitch, Roll and Yaw and cranial
adjustments (see Ch. 16) are also very important. Anyone
having problems on one side of the body, or some type of
asymmetry, is probably in need of integration.

Heart and Brain Integration "circuits" are often *not* "re-set,"
in the E.I., despite anti-fungal drugs, nutritional support and
avoidance of the "20th century." This is a central theme of this
book! But switching them on, and getting well, can be child's
play! The loss of brain and heart integration, often from formaldehyde and acetaldehyde (we hypothesize) causes the unfolding of downward spiraling health in the E.I. Neurological,
immunological, endocrinological and cardiovascular ills may
result. We also hope cardiologists will look at the use of this
exercise for their patients!

In 1985, the author extrapolated the concept of integration
beyond the brain and heart to include *all* the meridian/organ
systems.[49] These Rochlitz Meridian Integration Exercises are
beyond the scope here; they utilize the A.K./TFH muscle for
the appropriate meridian/organ system in analogous cross-
crawl fashion. See Fig. 23, where a kidney meridian integration
exercise is being performed. These have been taught in the
HEBS Seminars since 1985. They will appear in Vol. II.

Let's end our discussion of heart integration with another
discovery. We have realized that the connection of the heart to

Figure 23.

H.E.B.S. Kidney
Meridian
Integration
Exercise.

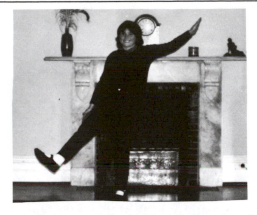

the muscle used in our corrective exercises is intuitively recognized by many societies and seems to be inherent in children. We've seen African tribal greeting and parting ceremonies. The dances contain arm waving that clearly uses the heart muscles. And how does a baby wave good-bye? Yes, it's from the heart! See Fig. 24.

Figure 24.

Saying good-bye from the heart.

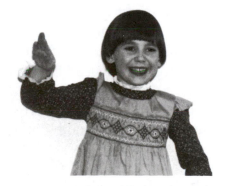

12

ENERGY BALANCING WITH KINESIOLOGY

Now we're ready to look at the rest of our breakthrough — the *PHYSICIST'S RAPID SOLUTION* — for allergy and Candida sufferers. Together with brain and heart integration and the other balancing methods of our "Psychology" chapter, the techniques of this chapter usually lead to a return of energy, balance, coordination, ability to read, think, concentrate and to be well in the E.I. It need not take years. (Often these are *never* regained, precisely because the methods of this book were unknown to those in the ecology field.) In many cases, this can happen in minutes. And if ecological vigilance is maintained in the short run, it will last. The body can then steadily recover and most people find that they can then begin to relax their ecological restrictions and still maintain wellness. Here we will study some simple techniques that can eliminate *energy imbalance* due to Candida, allergies and hypoglycemia. And you can do all these techniques on yourself! Remember, we are only saying that the energy imbalance from these disorders is corrected, we cannot claim that any disease is cured. You will have to find that out for yourself. Many thousands of people have found that they could not regain their health until these HEBS methods were performed.

Most of the methods in this chapter relate to what kinesiologists have called neurological disorganization in the body.[50] The sensitive feedback via MBT allows us to ascertain the status of neurological circuits unknown to the medical community. We have already touched on this idea in Ch. 9, where rubbing certain points helped normalize the body so MBT could then be used more accurately. Kinesiologists were the first to find ways of testing and correcting "circuits" that are used in maintaining coordination, balance, walking, seeing, hearing and other "reflexes." And this author was the first to realize that these corrections were needed because of ecological imbalance and that kinesiologists' corrections were often short-lived because the discoveries of clinical ecologists were not utilized simultaneously.

The first method we will examine is called *CLOACALS* or **CLOACAL RIGHTING REFLEXES**. Cloacal is the Latin word for sewer; it refers to the fact that lower animals have their eliminating and reproductive organs all located in one connected opening or canal. Animals, including ourselves, literally can't know "which end is up" unless the cloacal righting reflex is working properly. This reflex and the others in this chapter were apparently maintained in the higher animals even though there is more than "one canal." Many of these reflexes are crucial to maintaining *equilibrium* and relate to how the body knows where its major parts are. Some are in fact called "head on neck reflex," "labyrinth reflex," etc. We will present our own variations of these reflexes here.

As always, we need to know how to test and then correct this set of reflexes. But first we need to learn the "circuit lock" technique. (Advanced MBT methods use the terminology of electronics and computers!) All this lock does is free up the testor's hands, so he doesn't need to hold onto a point that tests weak. If you touch a point that makes a SIM go weak, you can "lock it in."

CIRCUIT LOCK TECHNIQUE

1. After checking that the muscle goes weak, hold (touch) the "weak" point or points.
2. Make sure the feet are touching each other for a moment.

3. Spread (abduct) the legs apart—straight out to the sides about 2-3 feet apart for most adults.

Then the testor can stop touching the weak point, but the imbalance should still be locked in weak! Muscle test to make sure. The massive hip *proprioceptors* are said to supply the memory that maintains the weak muscle response. (Proprioceptors gauge where the body's parts are in relation to each other. If they're not working properly, you will feel, and be, spaced out.) Each time you use the circuit lock (**CL**), you must first bring the legs together to erase any possible previous memories or inadvertent locks. Keep the legs apart for as long as you will be working with the particular imbalance. If you lose the lock, you will have to touch the weak point and lock it in, all over again.

Now we're ready for the front cloacals—see Fig. 25. (See also Fig. 27 for a view of front cloacal self-balancing.) Here we have two points that we will use as the "master testing points." These are points 1 and 2 and they are on the sides of the pubic bone. Find this bone in the pubic hair area. The points are an inch or so from the center (on each side).

FRONT CLOACAL TEST
1. Muscle test points 1 and 2 separately.
2. If either is weak, lock it in.
3. Check (test) that it is locked in weak.

FRONT CLOACAL CORRECTION
1. Next you will touch points 3, 4, 5, and 6 separately.
2. If any of these four points is part of the correction, at this time, it will make the weak lock become strong!
3. Points 3 and 4 you already know as the K27 points.
4. Points 5 and 6, perhaps the most important points on the front cloacals, are on the so-called supraorbital foramen. It is simply

a little notch in the bone *above* the eye. These points are a bit closer to the nose than the center of the eye is. Just feel along the bone until you find them. Now if point 1 is locked in weak and say points 4 and 6 separately cause the muscle to become strong, here's what you'll do.

5. The correction is a two-point, light holding, first of points 1 and 4 (for 20 seconds) and then points 1 and 6 (for 20 seconds).

6. In more detail, one hand (or really two fingers) will hold point 1 while the other hand touches point 4.

7. Likewise for points 1 and 6.

8. You can then retest. If it's corrected, the "weak" lock (of

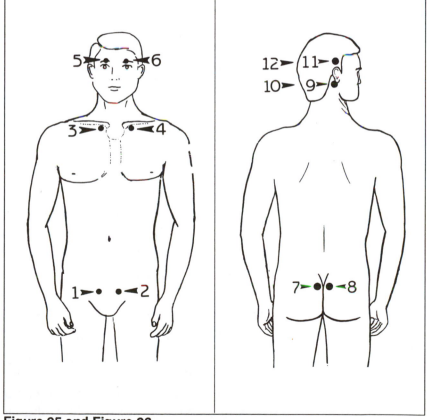

Figure 25 and Figure 26.
The front cloacals (left) and the back cloacals (right).

point 1) should now be strong.

9. Double check by putting the feet together and touch point 1; it should test strong.

The lock allows us to find which points will correct the weak point that is locked in. While touching each of the possible correcting points (3, 4, 5, and 6), remember that the one(s) that make the muscle go strong are the ones that are involved in correcting the weakness. If touching point 3 causes the locked in weakness of point 1 to remain weak, it is not involved and you can go on to see if the next possible correcting point does cause the muscle to go strong.

> **STOP READING NOW! YES, WE MEAN YOU! DO THIS SIMPLE CORRECTION NOW! DO IT, IF YOU WANT TO BE WELL. THERE ARE NO MAGIC PILLS THAT WILL GET YOU WELL! DON'T READ THIS BOOK LIKE A HISTORY BOOK – IT'S A SELF-HELP MANUAL. YES, YOU CAN DO THE CORRECTION EVEN WITHOUT TESTING IT. IT CAN'T HURT YOU! THE PHYSICIST'S RAPID SOLUTION WILL HAVE YOU FEELING BETTER ALMOST IMMEDIATELY AFTER YOU TAKE THESE FIRST STEPS.**

While lightly holding the points, you may feel the *capillary pulses* through your fingertips. You may even feel the pulses *synchronize*, telling you it's fixed; but this isn't crucial. While receiving the correction, some people feel a deep sense of relaxation, breathing may normalize and the stomach may gurgle as it "resets." Note that there are eight possible corrections on the front. Point 1 may have to be held (separately) with each of points 3, 4, 5, and 6. That's four possible corrections; and the same is true of point 2. That totals eight. (Chiropractic kinesiologists would do a similar set of corrections, except a very heavy pressing touch would be used. This would probably be painful. This may or may not be needed. Some have felt an even greater improvement, but correcting structural misalign-

ment cannot be our purpose here. Energy balancing is.)
The back side also has eight possible corrections. See Fig. 26.

BACK CLOACAL TEST

1. Here the master testing points are on the coccyx. (Points 7 and 8; the equivalent of 1 and 2 on the front.) The coccyx is the tailbone or the last vertebra of the spine. It's only an inch or so above the anus.
2. Each of these points is tested by going to the left (7) or right (8) of the coccyx, a fraction of an inch and pressing towards the center, lightly.
3. If points 7 or 8 tests weak, lock it in.

BACK CLOACAL CORRECTION

1. Now our set of possible correcting points are points 9, 10, 11, and 12.
2. Treat these four points as you treated points 3, 4, 5, and 6 on the front.
3. The correction is again a simultaneous two-point holding.

Points 9 and 10 are behind the ear, on the mastoid bone, just ¼ inch above where it comes to a tip behind the earlobe. One finger can be touching this point while the other finger touches the tip. Kinesiologists say this point is part of the body's labyrinth reflex. Points 11 and 12 are at slight indentations on the skull about an inch above the top of the ear and slightly behind the ear's center. You can cover this area with a large area of your four fingers to make sure you've got it. So test points 7 and 8. If weak, lock it in and see if touching points 9, 10, 11 and 12 make the locked muscle go strong.

The back cloacals are analogous to the front cloacals. Correcting cloacals together with brain integration exercises allowed the author to spin without dizziness for the first time in his life. This was performed by Joan Hulse in 1983. To my surprise, I immediately felt relaxed, energized and I found that I could perform spinning back (karate) kicks well for the first time.

> STOP READING NOW! YES, WE MEAN YOU! DO THIS SIMPLE CORRECTION NOW! DO IT, IF YOU WANT TO BE WELL. THERE ARE NO MAGIC PILLS THAT WILL GET YOU WELL! DON'T READ THIS BOOK LIKE A HISTORY BOOK – IT'S A SELF-HELP MANUAL. YES, YOU CAN DO THE CORRECTION EVEN WITHOUT TESTING IT. IT CAN'T HURT YOU! THE PHYSICIST'S RAPID SOLUTION WILL HAVE YOU FEELING BETTER ALMOST IMMEDIATELY AFTER YOU TAKE THESE FIRST STEPS.

The next technique is analogous to the cloacals and balances the region below the trunk as the cloacals balance the trunk itself. It is named after two German HEBS graduates.

MIX-WENZ TECHNIQUE
1. Here the master testing point is the bottom of the bone, i.e., the ball of the foot. (On each foot, of course.) It may hurt if pressed in. See Fig. 28 on the next page.
2. The set of possible correcting points are *now* the two pubic bone and the two coccyx points from before.

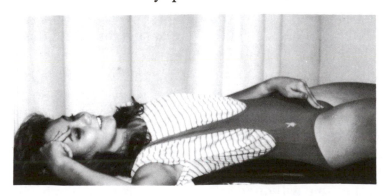

Figure 27. Self-correction of the cloacal righting reflexes.

3. So, if weak, lock in the ball of foot points and see which of the four possible correcting points is needed and
4. Perform the usual two hand touch correction.

STOP READING NOW! YES, WE MEAN YOU! DO THIS SIMPLE CORRECTION NOW! DO IT, IF YOU WANT TO BE WELL. THERE ARE NO MAGIC PILLS THAT WILL GET YOU WELL! DON'T READ THIS BOOK LIKE A HISTORY BOOK – IT'S A SELF-HELP MANUAL. YES, YOU CAN DO THE CORRECTION EVEN WITHOUT TESTING IT. IT CAN'T HURT YOU! THE PHYSICIST'S RAPID SOLUTION WILL HAVE YOU FEELING BETTER ALMOST IMMEDIATELY.

Those with a history of fungal toe nails or athlete's foot usually need this energy balance. Next we come to the HYOID correction which is related to maintaining brain integration. The hyoid

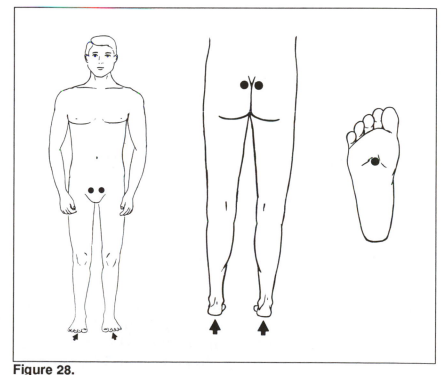

Figure 28.
Mix-Wenz Technique. The front points (left drawing), the back points (right) and the ball of foot.

is a "free-floating bone," behind and above the Adam's Apple, and held in place by 10 muscles. See Fig. 29. Some of these muscles also attach to the tongue. Problems with speech and frequent throat clearing are some signs of possible imbalance of the hyoid bone.

THE HYOID "SCREENING" TEST

1. Gently wiggle the hyoid bone left and right and in and out. (Reach around and behind the Adam's Apple.)
2. Quickly muscle test.
3. If weak, you need to know which muscles are too tight and how to relax them.
4. You can test each of these muscles by lightly "running" your fingers along each muscle in the figure.

We'll explain step #4 in detail now. Basically this includes running the muscle from under the center of the chin bone to the Adam's Apple, the muscle from the sternal notch up to the Adam's Apple, and four muscles diagonally towards the Adam's Apple as seen from the figure. This includes from the bottom left and right (starting at the outer third of the collar bone, on the left and right) and from the top left and right (near the edge of the jaw bone, under the ear). If running a muscle tests weak, it means that muscle is too tight.

We can correct it by the method known as *spindling* or spindle cell technique.

HYOID CORRECTION

1. Go to the *center* of the muscle(s) that tested weak and use the fingers of both hands to push *together* the fibers of the muscle.
2. Always push (or pinch together) along the direction that the fibers travel. See Fig. 29 again. If the fibers are vertical, your pushing together will be in a vertical direction. This spindling relaxes and lengthens the overtight muscles.

3. Retest the individual muscle by "running it" again.
4. When you're done, re-do the screening test. It should be strong.

Be gentle throughout – a karate technique is to quickly reach behind the Adam's Apple, grab and pull towards you. This can truly, permanently cure someone's allergies if you know what we mean. DON'T DO THIS!

The set of brain integration, cloacals, Mix-Wenz and hyoids seem to balance the body for imbalance due to Candida and aldehydes. Again they are not medical treatments; they can restore energy and wellness immediately and can't do any harm. This is just what the E.I. need (and what the doctor hasn't *yet* ordered).

There are more imbalances that need to be tested and corrected, however. GAIT REFLEXES are part of standing, walking and righting equilibrium and they can relate to brain integration. The test points are between the toe bones, less than an inch below where the toes join the feet. As Fig. 30 indicates,

Figure 29.

Hyoids with spindling shown.

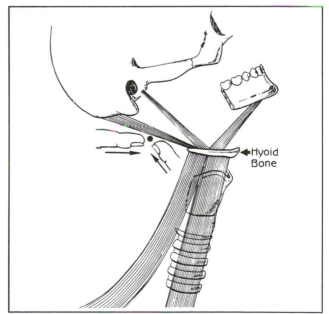

there are also test points to the side of the bones coming from the pinky and big toes and at the ball of the foot. Your test pressure will be a bit heavier than the earlier pressures used.

GAIT REFLEXES

1. If a gait point tests weak (when touched),
2. The correction is a heavy rubbing at this point or points. You can rub them all to be sure.

This may hurt and make this clear to the subject. He should always have the option of saying, "no thanks." Of course a central theme of this book is that the corrections herein are designed so that *you* can do them all on *yourself*! And there is a behavioral factor; it almost always hurts *less* when you do the pressing or rubbing on yourself! (Similarly, you won't feel tickled either, if you do this yourself.) On the other hand, some would say that especially for the gentle holding, energy corrections, having someone else send in some energy is a good idea and lets you relax and enjoy the correction or balance. Though the gait corrections may hurt, you should feel a great increase

Figure 30.

Gait reflex points. Add the ball of the foot (not shown).

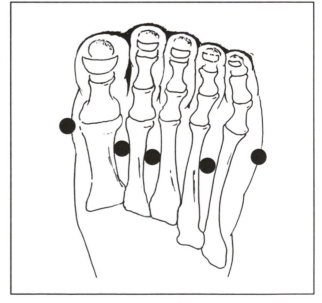

in energy and athletic ability! Gait reflexes going out and much leg and even back pain may be due to *Morton's Neuroma*. This is a growth of the nerve ending between the second and third smallest toes. It is largely unknown or misunderstood by physicians except for podiatrists.

STOP READING NOW! YES, WE MEAN YOU! DO THIS SIMPLE CORRECTION NOW! DO IT, IF YOU WANT TO BE WELL. THERE ARE NO MAGIC PILLS THAT WILL GET YOU WELL! DON'T READ THIS BOOK LIKE A HISTORY BOOK—IT'S A SELF-HELP MANUAL. YES, YOU CAN DO THE CORRECTION EVEN WITHOUT TESTING IT. IT CAN'T HURT YOU! THE PHYSICIST'S RAPID SOLUTION WILL HAVE YOU FEELING BETTER ALMOST IMMEDIATELY AFTER YOU TAKE THESE FIRST STEPS.

Now let's come to more advanced testing and corrections for poor balance and spatial confusion. Again this is known as **PITCH, ROLL AND YAW** or **PRY**. The testing and corrections from Chapter 9 are less powerful and shorter-lived than the ones here. PRY refers to neurological disorganization in the body. The brain and structure (cranium and spine) are not functioning properly. This is a tremendous energy drain on the body. (Medicine will hopefully acknowledge this soon.) Pitch refers to a confusion between top and bottom. Some of the nerve signals meant for the right *biceps* might go to the right *quadriceps*. Roll refers to a left-right disorganization. Some signals meant for the *right* biceps might go to the *left* biceps. And Yaw is a front-back disorganization. Some energy meant for the right *biceps* might go to the right *triceps*.

These tests were devised by Goodheart, his corrections were primarily chiropractic adjustments and so can't be given here. Instead we primarily use the corrections devised by Richard Utt.[51]

PITCH TEST

1. Start out with the subject lying flat and facing up.
2. Have him/her bring the knees up with the feet on the floor (or table)

3. Muscle test this. If weak, have him roll into a ball and roll on his hip bones to correct them. (If still not strong, see your chiropractic physician.)

4. Next bring the feet back straight out as they were at first.

5. Bring the head up, chin towards the chest and test this. If weak, massage the neck or see a chiropractor and/or a massage therapist.

6. *The actual test for the Pitch is to bring the knees up and the head up simultaneously.* This is why we had to make sure the two were first strong separately. If one were out we couldn't accurately test the two positions together which is the actual Pitch test. (See Fig. 31.) If Pitch is out, we can correct as follows.

PITCH CORRECTION

This and the ROLL and YAW corrections are a bit advanced; do them only if you're comfortable working with the body. The feet are lying flat during the corrections. Place one hand on the subject's forehead and the other against the bottom of his head. The correction will involve the subject's head and chin coming up (towards his chest) while you push down with the hand on his forehead (but not enough to stop him from coming up) and

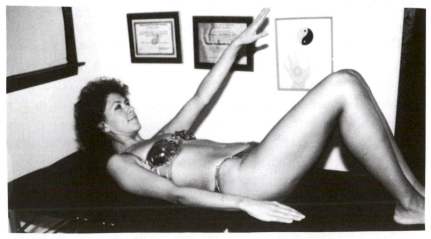

Figure 31. Testing position for the Pitch "computer."

the subject going back down while you apply upwards pressure with your bottom hand. Each motion lasts for about two seconds in each direction. Do it about seven times unless the subject gets exhausted. You can prevent this by offering the following advice. Make sure the subject is not holding his breath. Remind him to breathe in and out deeply and slowly throughout these corrections. Watch that he is not straining facial and neck muscles, as many are prone to do. Most people make these corrections tough on themselves with all sorts of conditioned straining. And yes, all the PRY corrections here can be done all by yourself, if need be! Just use your own hands.

A retest should now be strong. There are some experiential changes that you can also check for. Remember Pitch refers to top-to-bottom switching or neurological disorganization. In some people, the stretch, straight to the toes, is noticeably improved. Demonstrate before and after either from a standing or lying position and note the difference. In some, fear of heights is corrected. If not, it's a true emotional phobia and the answer lies in Ch. 15. Also many with this imbalance write their n's and h's alike and this can be fixed with this correction.

Now we're ready for the ROLL.

ROLL TEST

1. The test is to bring the knees up and place the feet near the buttocks as before.

2. Only now let the knees hang all the way over to the left (for the left Roll) and all the way over to the right (for the right Roll). These hip positions are tested separately (while the head is on the table) and must be strong. If not, do some rolling around on the hips.

3. The actual left and right Roll tests are to have the knees over as stated and to bring the head up to the same position as in the Pitch test. The corrections are as follows.

ROLL CORRECTION

If the left Roll was weak (chin to the chest and knees to the left), turn the head all the way to the left and have the testor place one hand on the top (right temple) and his other hand on the bottom (left temple) of the subject's head. There will be the same up and down motion *against* the testor's hands as with the Pitch correction. Only here the head must at all times remain facing to the side that is being corrected. I.e., turned to the left as it comes up and down for the left Roll correction; and turned to the right throughout the right Roll correction. Watch, and correct for, straining and breath-holding as before. Do seven or eight up and down motions. (See Fig. 32.)

Retest the weak Roll(s). They should now be strong. Experiential tests are as follows. Before the correction, have the subject remain in the vertical plane throughout, but have him bend towards the left and right sides. Mark (against his pants) with chalk, the lowest point that the middle finger can reach on the left and right. There should be a noticeable difference in the heights of left and right stretches. They should even up; i.e., one should come up and the other down after the correction(s). Also

Figure 32.

Correcting the Right Roll. (Head pushes up against the top hand; and pushes down against bottom hand.)

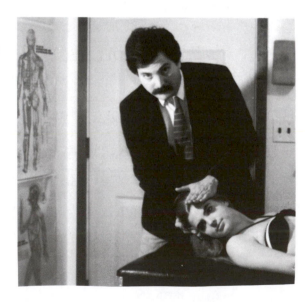

the classic dyslexic mix-up between p's and q's and b's and d's may be improved. But brain integration may have already corrected this. We have found an intricate connection between brain integration and the Roll or left-to-right neurological (dis)organization. Some people will also spin better after this correction, but for others, the Yaw must first be corrected.

Here's how we test and correct the YAW "computer."

YAW TEST

1. The knees will be in the same position as in the Roll tests.

2. Only here the head is raised and turned to the *opposite* direction of the knees. We will define left and right as the direction of the knees. Thus the left Yaw test is to have the knees raised and over to the left while the head is raised and turned to the right. Test after attaining the position.

3. The right Yaw test reverses the head and leg positions.

YAW CORRECTION

There is one tricky element to the corrections here. The head must face in the direction that the *knees* (and not the head) were. So for the left Yaw correction, the head will turn to the left, not the right as it was in the actual, left Yaw test. Thus, correct left Yaw by having the head facing to the left and moving *toward and away* from the left shoulder (and back to the center). You needn't have the head raised, it can be resting against the table as it moves towards and away from the shoulder. The testor's hands are against the forehead and the back of the head to facilitate the usual resistance. As always, the subject can actually do these corrections on himself.

When Yaw is corrected many can safely spin and others stop bumping into walls and other objects as they walk.

A good before-and-after test is to have the subject sit up

and place his feet flat against the floor with the feet spread apart. Stretch the left hand to the right leg and note the distance. Likewise for the right hand to the left leg. Note any differences before and after the corrections. Sometimes the straightforward stretch only improves after all PRY corrections are made. Also with these PRY corrections from Utt, some feel their vertebrae "pop" back into place. These are priceless corrections for your balance, equilibrium, energy and health. Your brain and structure have been corrected!

Next we come to a correction that has been dubbed "BLOOD CHEMISTRY CORRECTION" by kinesiologists. We can make no claims for this, but have interviewed people who said their lives were saved by this correction. This circuit may also be out of balance from something as simple as faulty blood sugar which can come as a reaction to eating the wrong food or from *not* eating! See Fig. 33.

BLOOD CHEMISTRY ENERGY TEST

1. The test is to touch each Sp21 (Spleen 21) point. This point, is on the ribs where the inside elbow crease intersects them. This is really on the meridian that relates to the pancreas.
2. If weak, lock it in.

BLOOD CHEMISTRY ENERGY CORRECTION

1. Find which of the K27 points (when touched, while in the lock) makes the weak arm become strong.
2. The correction is a two-hand, simultaneous tapping with moderate pressure (one hand tapping a Sp21 point and the other hand simultaneously tapping a K27 point). Unfortunately, as always, if a point is imbalanced, it's often painful.
3. Tap 30 times. You can even tap with a harmonizing waltz beat — HARD-soft-soft. (If unsure, you can always tap all four possible corrections.)
4. Retest; it should now be O.K.

STOP READING NOW! YES, WE MEAN YOU! DO THIS SIMPLE CORRECTION NOW! DO IT, IF YOU WANT TO BE WELL. THERE ARE NO MAGIC PILLS THAT WILL GET YOU WELL! DON'T READ THIS BOOK LIKE A HISTORY BOOK – IT'S A SELF-HELP MANUAL. YES, YOU CAN DO THE CORRECTION EVEN WITHOUT TESTING IT. IT CAN'T HURT YOU! THE PHYSICIST'S RAPID SOLUTION WILL HAVE YOU FEELING BETTER ALMOST IMMEDIATELY AFTER YOU TAKE THESE FIRST STEPS.

Clearly this is a Spleen (pancreas)-Kidney Meridian communication correction. But it can reset faulty blood sugar (energy) imbalances and more serious abnormalities. No, it's not

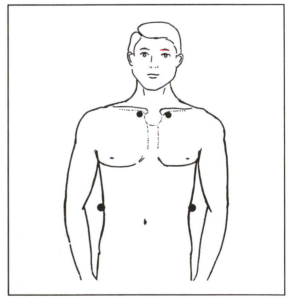

Figure 33.

"Blood Chemistry Energy Correction."

Often helpful for hypoglycemics.

permanent. This always depends on your ecology and other factors.

Let's look at a simple correction that can help normalize intestinal functioning via energy balancing. This correction is for the two intestinal valves, the ILEOCECAL (IC) VALVE (on the right side) and the HOUSTON VALVE (on the left). The ileocecal valve is at the junction of the end of the small intestine and the beginning of the large intestine. It's about half way between the navel and the protruding, front hip bone near the side (the ASIS). The Houston valve separates two regions of the colon. It's at a similar location on the left side. The ileocecal valve is almost always "switched off" in the E.I. If there are underlying overgrowths, the correction may have to be performed many times. (Killing overgrowths may be necessary.) It's possible that overgrowths of parasites or C.a. may exist on the valve itself. The Houston valve imbalance is less frequently found. These valves can be either (too) open or closed. The open condition refers to a valve that is flaccid and can't completely close. The closed condition refers to spastic or overtight valve muscles.

If you have diarrhea or constipation, this energy balance could help. See Fig. 34 for the corrections. One set of corrections will fix either valve whether it is in the open or closed condition.

ILEOCECAL & HOUSTON VALVE CORRECTION

1. There are three sets of (light) two-point holding corrections.
2. Do all three sets on one side then do the other side
3. Hold the two points labeled 1 for 20 seconds.
4. Then hold the second set of points similarly before completing the balance with the third set.

> **STOP READING NOW! YES, WE MEAN YOU! DO THIS SIMPLE CORRECTION NOW! DO IT, IF YOU WANT TO BE WELL. THERE ARE NO MAGIC PILLS THAT WILL GET YOU WELL! DON'T READ THIS BOOK LIKE A HISTORY BOOK – IT'S A SELF-HELP MANUAL. YES, YOU CAN DO THE CORRECTION EVEN WITHOUT TESTING IT. IT CAN'T HURT YOU! THE PHYSICIST'S RAPID SOLUTION WILL HAVE YOU FEELING BETTER ALMOST IMMEDIATELY.**

You can do this several times a day. For some people, these valves go "out" as soon as they cheat on their diet.

Finally we will learn how to *RESET OUR EYES AND EARS*.

Now, for the EYES, if focusing on a spot tests weak, or you simply feel eye strain, do the following.

RESET OR "SWITCH ON" THE EYES

1. With your hands outstretched in front of you, clasp the fingers.
2. Trace the so-called "lazy 8." (It's an eight so lazy, it's lying on its back. Some of us though would call it an infinity sign.) Tracing means you look *only* at your outstretched hands (and not the room or your testor!) as they follow the lazy 8 pattern.
3. Always start by going over your *top left*; see the double arrow in Fig. 35. This exercise can help re-integrate your eyes.

Figure 34.

Ileocecal and Houston Valve Correction Points.

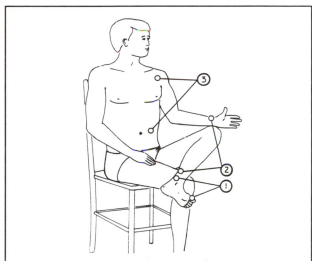

4. If any dizziness results, it probably means you need Pitch, Roll and Yaw correction — go to it!

Lastly, we will test and correct our *EARS*. This test is a bit different as follows.

"SWITCHED OFF" EAR TEST

1. With the subject looking straight ahead, block off the ear as follows.

2. Place a flat palm an inch or two out from the ear and muscle test.

3. This should be weak! This is because, from Eastern medicine, the ears are actually antennae that pick up energy. When blocked off, this is weakening. However, if the ears are "switched off" in the first place, there is no circuit functioning to go weak, so the arm remains strong.

4. So, if the arm tests *strong*, the ear is switched off and must be corrected.

SWITCHING ON THE EARS

1. The correction, see Fig. 36, is to unravel (radially outward) the outer part of the ear, going completely around (clockwise) as you unravel.

2. Do this five times.

3. Retest; the arm should now go *weak* meaning the ear is now switched on and doesn't like being blocked off!

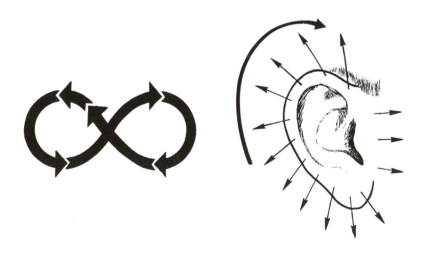

Figure 35 and Figure 36.
Switching on the eyes, Fig. 35 (left) and ears, Fig. 36 (right).

STOP READING NOW! YES, WE MEAN YOU! DO THIS
SIMPLE CORRECTION NOW! DO IT, IF YOU WANT
TO BE WELL. THERE ARE NO MAGIC PILLS THAT
WILL GET YOU WELL! DON'T READ THIS BOOK
LIKE A HISTORY BOOK – IT'S A SELF-HELP
MANUAL. YES, YOU CAN DO THE CORRECTION
EVEN WITHOUT TESTING IT. IT CAN'T HURT YOU!
THE PHYSICIST'S RAPID SOLUTION WILL HAVE
YOU FEELING BETTER ALMOST IMMEDIATELY
AFTER YOU TAKE THESE FIRST STEPS.

This can be a powerful energy boost as the points on the ear
also relate to meridians and chakras (nerve plexus). This often
also helps relieve some neck pain or tension. The ears can
switch off on their own, or from loud or bad sounds, or from
sleeping on the wrong side. This simple correction can be
performed twice a day, as can any other correction in this book,
if need be. Boost your energies now!

We often ask a new client to spin before doing any corrections.
Only after correcting brain and heart integration, "Figure 8"
imbalance (See Ch. 15), hyoids, cloacals, PRY, "blood
chemistry correction," eyes and ears – do we ask the client to
spin again. Most of the time it is vastly improved, with many
saying it's the first time in their lives that they can spin! Again
this is why we have called the condition of car sickness and
trouble riding a merry-go-round in childhood, "pre-Candidiasis
imbalance." Nearly all adults with long-term E.I. that we've
asked have said that they had these complaints as *children*. Thus
long before the serious chemical imbalances manifested, significant "electrical" imbalance occurred. It's always a joy to
correct these imbalances in children, thus preventing a lifetime
of suffering. Also it strengthens the immune system, helping to
nip E.I. in the bud. (A yeast joke.)

For some people, some of these corrections need be done only
once to notice remarkable changes in their health. These
people we say are suffering *more from the ELECTROMAG-
NETIC HARMFUL EFFECTS OF CANDIDA, ALDEHYDES,*

PARASITES, etc. and *less* from chemical imbalance! We can't stress this enough. It's an entire Universe missing from the ecologists' picture and is why so many with E.I. go on suffering after anti-fungal drugs, supplementation and "avoidance of the 20th century." And why thousands have gotten well very rapidly now, around the world, from the HEBS system of balancing energy and ecology. This author always knew there had to be a better way or at least an additional fork in the road — as these methods are complementary, not mutually exclusive. For others with *tremendous* overgrowths, these corrections may need to be done several times a day to maintain some degree of wellness. Don't let this phase you — do your balancing as needed. We assert that for virtually everyone with E.I., the energy balancing can significantly compress the time needed to overcome E.I. In the short run, diet and environmental restrictions should also be followed. And realize that there are many more balancing methods and options available to eclectic kinesiologists at this time. The total corrections available to kinesiologists could fill not just a chapter or a book, but an entire library!

A word now on the author's 1983 discovery of the so-called *"CANDIDA BALANCE."*[53] This is what got the author well, in less than five minutes! We usually say an hour as most wouldn't believe 32 years of suffering could be halted in minutes, but it was. The Candida balance has been borrowed by other kinesiologies and altered (and may not be effective — we can take no responsibility for this). This balance refers to the amazing fact that, on an individual basis, Candida and aldehyde energy imbalance can be locked in and corrected in so-called priority fashion. This methodology is more effective, safer, less interactive and much more rapid than methods like neutralization from the clinical ecologists. Some of the methods we use are based on the great, pioneering kinesiologist, Alan Beardall, D.C. Here MBT is used as changes in skin cell electrical conductivity[54] (lie detector) could, to tell the testor what circuits have been switched off in the individual and even how to optimally correct them. You know that a lie detector can gauge the body's response to something as "esoteric" as a thought.

With the most advanced balancing methods, the techniques of this chapter may be needed or they may be corrected intrinsically! Meridians, muscles, emotions, nutrition, chakras[55] may all be balanced as called for by the body's memory! Often many chemical and pollen (along with some food) sensitivities are corrected in an hour of balancing. The food allergies remaining can then be locked in and many can be similarly balanced. This is the most powerful and beneficial type of balancing. It is somewhat analogous to homeopathy. In homeopathy — a 150 year old medical science — deep healing is performed via a very diluted constitutional remedy. (Difficulties arise with homeopathic remedies for the E.I. They are in sucrose, lactose or alcohol bases.) This is, in effect, individualized energy balancing. Only homeopathy depends on an external prescriber to figure out the remedy. In advanced MBT, the body itself — when asked properly — will say what it needs. But it is impossible to teach this in a book. We do have certified instructors around the world. And the methods in this chapter will get you well! If need be, you can re-balance yourself everyday, until it's no longer necessary. But remember the HEBS methods are not panaceas.

However, it is one of the central themes of this book that many with Candida overgrowth are functioning well (for the time being) precisely because they have not (yet) had the "switches," described in this chapter, switched off. (See Fig. 37.) We've seen many with coated tongues and GI complaints that seemed well. Sure enough, when tested they still had these switches working properly. We can't stress this point enough and hope the ecologists add this other half of the puzzle to their conceptualization. This is not to deny the significance of the research on the "chemical" aspects of E.I. But, nature has revealed that only energy *and* ecology vigilance and balancing works!

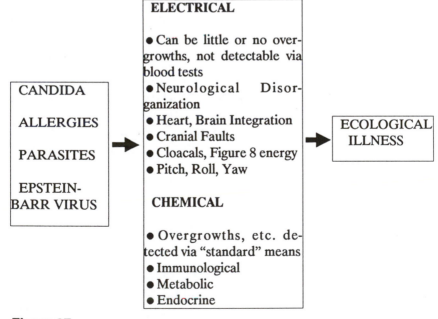

Figure 37.
Towards a complete picture of Ecological Illness (and Kinesiology).

13

ECOLOGICAL NUTRITION

Now we're ready to have a unique study of nutrition specifically geared for the Ecologically Ill. Ecological considerations usually override nutritional ones and this is often not recognized by many nutritionists. As always, kinesiological testing allows for truly individualized nutritional support. In this chapter, we will detail special tips on how to eat, as well as, recent breakthroughs in nutrition. These include essential fatty acid metabolism, B6 metabolism, vitamin phosphorylation and amino acid metabolism. We won't discuss what all the vitamins and minerals do, as this information is readily available in your book store, health food store or medical library. If you are unfamiliar with vitamins and minerals, make it a point to inspect several books on this topic and read *one* that you like. The HEBS system is the only wellness system in the world that covers ecology, nutrition, kinesiology and integration.

It is wise to understand our human tendencies and weaknesses. We may want only to study more of the field(s) we already have some expertise in. This tendency should be fought. Please make it a point to study those fields that you are *least* adept at (of the four), instead of just getting better at the one(s) you already know!

EATING TIPS

We begin by repeating some of the "obvious." Avoid allergic foods. Continually test yourself as allergies change. Avoid eating safe foods too frequently as they may become allergenic. See Appendix C if you want to use a rotary diversified diet. Don't eat when under physical or emotional stress. Do eat after de-stressing yourself with ESR (see Ch. 15) or meditation. Eat in ecologically sound environments. Have good air, lighting, music, friends and other ambient conditions. Avoid electric watches, LCD's, TV's, etc. Eat, and go outdoors during the day. You can eat shortly after exercising as this often prevents reactions unless you are in the stressful building-up phase of exercising.

Don't overeat as many Americans do. This can stress your detoxifying organs and actually lead to malnourishment. Avoid the four classes of foods that may favor Candidiasis. These are simple carbohydrates, foods with molds, allergens, and foods with free radicals, especially oily or fried foods. You will probably be eating a lot of fish and vegetables. If you don't like the idea, then these are probably good foods for you! You must also be careful not to eat too much meat. This, in effect, will have you ingesting too high a percentage of your calories from protein and fat. Your kidneys and gall bladder, respectively, would be stressed if you overeat meats.Try to get most of your calories from complex carbohydrates (starchy foods) that you can eat.

As most of the allergy or Candida cook books (that we have seen) have recipes with heated oils (or other contradictions), we can't recommend one yet. But shortly, several HEBS graduates have indicated they will have good cook books written and we will then make these available.

If you are hypoglycemic (which may self-correct if you do everything appropriate), eat frequent, small meals. This also is less stressful to the digestive system. Don't drink while eating as this dilutes the enzymes. Do drink plenty of good water 45 minutes before and an hour after eating. Drink at least eight glasses of water a day. Chemically and kinesiologically test your water. Muscle test water from a purifier, if possible, before purchase. Always be on guard for new cravings. Chew your food very well. Avoid raw or undercooked meats and fish. Avoid foods with artificial ingredients, rancid elements or foods that may have been "left over" too long. Avoid foods that have a high surface area of exposure for molds and bacteria, like chopped meats. Eat a very high fiber diet with lots of green vegetables. If advised, take your digestive enzymes at the beginning of the meal. Alkaline bicarbonates can be taken 45-60 minutes after the meal along with any amino acid supplements. The bicarbonates would be needed if the intestines are not alkaline enough or to combat systemic over-acidity, if present.

Be aware that nutritional supplements may be best absorbed if *chewed*, instead of swallowed. This is the natural way that the body has for ascertaining what nutrients are being ingested. It can thus make appropriate enzymes. Some of the nutrient may also be absorbed, into the blood, from under the tongue. Also if a nutrient is poorly absorbed, taking it alone may improve its absorption as there is *competition* between similar nutrients (as with a multivitamin-mineral). You can have your digestive enzymes tested. One way is by your physician's use of the Heidelberg capsule. You swallow this and it telemeters — to an electronic device — your GI pH (acid-alkaline state) as it traverses your tract. You can also buy pH paper from your laboratory supply company (in the yellow pages). Saliva pH supposedly mirrors intestinal pH and should be around 7.5. Urine pH mirrors the stomach's pH, and it (the urine) should be around 5.5. (The elderly and many with E.I. are often put on antacids when in fact they need to *augment* low stomach acidity which allows things to ferment and cause pain.) Don't over-take nutrients.

Correct these as needed with your nutritionist's advice. Be wary of books that recommend many hundreds of milligrams of B-vitamins. Note that, for some people, excess nutrients, e.g. iron, biotin, other B-vitamins, zinc may lead to yeast over-growth. The bacterially-derived B-vitamins must also be tested. All these nutrients may be needed, at some time, in smaller amounts, as blood and other tests indicate. You can never be tested too much!

Avoid excess sodium. Though not an allergy, it can lead to edema, weather sensitivity, neurological and neuromuscular symptoms, dehydration, and has even been linked to cancer. Craving salt may be a sign of adrenal exhaustion. Avoid eating out — cooks and waiters may not be honest about ingredients. Cook and serve food only in glass, porcelain, cast iron and stainless steel. Avoid the last two, if you are metal-sensitive. Test your toothpaste and anything else that goes down the hatch or on your person or that you breathe. (Also test lighting, sounds, and any other ambient energies.)

Do learn, and abide by, *FOOD COMBINING* guidelines. See Fig. 38. Basically fruits should be eaten alone. Likewise for heavy protein or fatty foods. You may be able to get away with some complex carbohydrate at the same meal. Test this experientially as some cannot. You can eat green vegetables with almost anything. Get a book or carry-card on food combining from your health food store and study it. Eat according to the present state of your biological clock — see Ch. 16. If the weather conditions are bothering you, consider eating very little, at the time. If you will not be at home, have safe foods prepared *ahead of time*. Avoid cheating binges. Don't hate yourself if one starts, just get back on track. Consider fasting and colonics (first consult a knowledgeable physician) to rest your digestive and eliminating organs. This author has fasted

---

Non-starchy & green vegetables — goes with any food
includes: green leafy veggies, cabbage, lettuce, celery, etc.
Starchy vegetables — with green salad, not with protein or fruit
includes: potato, corn, squash, coconut, artichoke, carrot
Proteins — with salads, not with starch or fruits
includes: meats, sprouts, beans, nuts, seeds, grains
Melons — alone, or avoid if have Candida
Sub-acid fruits — only with either acid or sweet fruits
includes: papaya, mango, apple, pear, cherry, berries, grapes, peach
Acid fruits — only with sub-acid fruits
includes: citrus, pineapple, strawberries, pomegranate
Sweet fruits — only with sub-acid fruits or celery & lettuce
includes: banana, carob, dates

Figure 38. Food Combining Guidelines.

for 14 days (just water) on several occasions.

Test and correct your *ACID-ALKALINE BALANCE* as follows. (This test is derived from John Diamond, M.D.) See Fig. 39.

ACID-ALKALINE ENERGY TEST

1. First find out if the subject is right-handed or not.

2. If right handed, have him hold up (vertically) his flat (right) palm 2 inches away from the right temple. (Don't block the ear.)

3. Test with his left arm.

4. If weak, an over-acid condition supposedly exists.

5. Take his right arm and have him block off his left temple.

6. If his (left) arm tests weak, an over-alkaline condition exists.

7. Now for the lefties.

8. The dominant hand does the blocking again. But here that's the left. The muscle tested here will be the right.

9. If the left hand covers the left temple and the right arm tests weak, an over-acid condition may exist.

10. And if the left hand covering the right temple tests weak, an over-alkaline condition may exist.

Figure 39.

Acid-Alkaline Test.

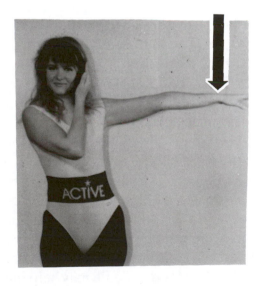

These results supposedly refer to systemic and not GI conditions. We note that allergic reactions can lead to a systemic acid condition (acidosis). Arthritics are usually too acid. Taking alkaline salts an hour after eating can reverse such a trend. Hopefully avoiding allergens will lead to self-correction.

Dietary and supplement corrections may help correct these imbalances. If too acid, alkalinizing foods are needed. This would include many fruits and vegetables. (Citrus and tomatoes are excluded.) Correct over-alkalinity with grains and meats. These create acid conditions. See your food-combining book for further suggestions!

Be aware that most supplements can be allergenic. You can rotate supplements as you do foods. Consider frequent halts to your supplement regimen just in case the MBT misses something. Never put all your stock in only one modality (including MBT). Watch out for overeating of proteins and fats as these are usually the "safest foods." You can use a nutrition almanac to gauge the amount of fat, say, in your diet.

The nutrient *RNA* is said to be an overall circuit booster. Unfortunately, many kinesiologists used to test and recommend yeast-containing RNA supplements. A better source is a thymus glandular extract which also contains immune factors. Test this too. Test nutrients only with the HEBS methods. (Using a tiny piece, here.) Chewing and testing should be avoided — it's inaccurate. This is also true of supplement testing as noted earlier. Consider vitamin injections, if needed; but test them as they may contain toxic or allergenic preservatives. You may not need injections if underlying factors (like overgrowths and enzyme deficiencies) are corrected. Get a hair analysis and look for heavy metal toxicities. Most hair analyses are accurate for lead, copper and other heavy metal excesses. Be aware that the temperature of food can affect you and your metabolism. Cold food or liquid may help you to sleep as it helps make the hormone-neurotransmitter, serotonin, from the amino acid, tryptophane. Hot food or liquid may help make other hormones from tyrosine.

Though we recommend nutritional support, this should never be done unconditionally. Though far less dangerous than drugs, there are points to be made aware of. We will first list some "con's" And then the "pro's."

CON'S OF NUTRITIONAL SUPPLEMENTATION

Here, we present the worst possible, hypothetical scenarios. Many supplements are allergenic. (Avoid any companies that claim to be "non-allergenic"—a sure sign of ignorance or fraud.) Many are spoiled or rancid. Most of the hypoallergenic companies are not manufacturers, but are distributors. This means the nutrients are around longer before they get to your stomach. Nutrients can oxidize or go rancid easily. This includes the anti-oxidant nutrients too. E.g., Vit. C. (ascorbic acid) oxidizes to dehydroascorbic acid which is toxic. The pancreas may preferentially be affected. If your Vit. C powder becomes yellow instead of white, get rid of it.

Supplements may be shelved for long periods in stores too. Some large distributors have very low prices, but use the manufacturer's *rejects*. As is usually the case, you get what you pay for. Many allow supplements to spoil by letting them sit too long or allowing them to heat up or get too cold. If you test weak to a supplement, get rid of it. Because this illness has been financially devastating—until this book!—many hold onto their allergenic supplements in the hope they'll be O.K. some time later. Don't.

The author has seen many clients who have flown in from around the world. MBT often reveals their worst problem is allergenic supplements, usually medically recommended without any way of testing for allergies. Many companies use American overkill. While their capsules may have one or two safe nutrients, the company feels they have to be "one up" on their competition; so they add an additional dozen ingredients.

This virtually guarantees something in the capsule will be a problem for many people! Less can definitely be more here. Get only what you need. Another frequent allergic supplement is the pervasive adrenal glandular tablet or capsule. Some "holistic" practitioners hand this out to most of their patients in analogous fashion to the way the orthodox physician uses cortisone drugs to fight stress or illness when they don't really know what is happening. Most people are, or soon become, allergic to the adrenal glandulars. Learn MBT and you can save both a fortune and your health.

Some nutritional kinesiologists find their Candida clients only get well when *taken off* most or all supplements, especially B-vitamins. (Some people can also have trouble getting to sleep from taking excess B-vitamins.) It is also possible to develop some sort of tolerance and dependence on vitamins. The body does this with Vit. C. Infants born to mothers who were taking large doses of Vit. C develop a sort of "rebound scurvy" as would anyone who suddenly stops taking this vitamin. There are two general reasons that supplements can become a problem. You already know the first—they're taken everyday. The second possibility is uniquely revealed here. Recall that we have mentioned the science of homeopathy where substances become very potent when diluted and succussed (shaken). This, to an extent, may happen in the manufacture of supplements. Finally some would say that taking supplements is just plain unnatural.

Now for the counterpoint—the benefits of nutritional supplementation.

PRO'S OF NUTRITIONAL SUPPLEMENTATION

First, once you know the cons, you can counteract them. E.g., cut back slowly on Vit. C, instead of doing it all at once. The need for Vit. C can be clearly manifested. A darker (than usual) urine color may indicate, you've taken more than enough.

Under stress, such as from a cold, a much higher dose would be required to see this color in the urine. You can take up to this threshold amount. Now, in more general terms, a nutritional deficiency may be at the root of a medical condition or sub-clinical complaint. Sensitivity to Monosodium Glutamate (MSG) can be due to a lack of the P5P form of Vitamin B6 (see below) and sulfite sensitivity can be due to a deficiency of molybdenum. (Of course, the parasite/permeability factors may always be the earliest causes allowing large amounts of these toxic substances to enter the blood.) Thus wellness cannot be attained *without* supplementation. Hypoallergenic supplements may be obtainable. They can even be rotated. You can get single item supplements if you look. Less can be more! There is hardly any life-threatening dangers to supplementing, unlike pharmaceutical prescribing. Drugs, not vitamins, have LD-50's. (Lethal dose at which 50% of experimental animals will die.) Emotional and physical stress have been proven to deplete nutrients.

Most foods eaten are deficient in many nutrients for the following reasons: Abuse and overuse of the soil, use of fertilizers, pesticides, freezing, canning and processing of food, loss during transportation, loss during cooking. How many eat only organic foods just plucked from the ground as nature intended? Certain crucial microminerals like molybdenum and selenium are almost completely depleted from the soil. Yes, the pro's outweigh the con's. Some say supplementation leads to expensive urine and is thus a waste. But who would say paying insurance premiums for your house is a waste because it hasn't yet burned down! And expensive urine is a lot cheaper than paying for the expensive physicians that say such things to their patients.

Recall some of our previous discussions had much nutritional relevance. Chapter 11 listed cardiovascular supporting nutrients. Chapter 6 listed the food sources of supplements. Chapter 7 listed anti-aldehyde and anti-fungal nutrients. On the next page, we list anti-oxidant nutrients.

ANTI-OXIDANTS

Vitamin A
Vitamin C
Vitamin E
Vitamins $B_{1,2,3,5,6}$, B_{15} (or N,N Dimethylglycine), PABA
Bioflavonoids
Selenium
Zinc
Superoxide dismutase (SOD)
Glutathione
Cysteine.

The anti-oxidants either directly scavenge free radicals or they are nutrients that are incorporated into enzymes that perform this task. E.g., glutathione is part of the glutathione peroxidase enzyme that detoxifies the dangerous lipid peroxide *radicals* found in all heated oils and in other substances. Free radicals are *highly reactive* substances. They have an unpaired electron, and by the laws of physics are desperate to find another electron by attaching to anything. The free radical can damage any molecule or cell that it attaches to. Free radical damage was known for some time to be part of aging theory. And more recently, it has been found to be a large part of the misery of the E.I. Allergic reactions already create many free radicals. You don't need to get them (already formed) from your diet. In this light, some nutritionists assert that nearly all nuts sold in America are rancid. The fats have gone bad — they've oxidized or become free radicals.

Let's begin to discuss several recent advances in nutrition. As always here, we gear this discussion to the E.I. This may be most people who take supplements whether they realize this or not. **VITAMIN B6** may be the most important vitamin for the E.I. We list some of the functions of B_6. It's needed for amino acid metabolism — thus to form hormones, neurotransmitters, enzymes, antibodies, red blood cells, etc. It's needed in fatty acid

and carbohydrate metabolism and for cardiovascular metabolism and proper neurological functioning. It can reduce edema,
help make stomach acid and help Vit. B_{12} absorption.

NEEDED FOR PROPER B_6 METABOLISM
Magnesium
Zinc
Cysteine
Other B-Vitamins like B_2
Citric acid (made by the body, not from citrus fruits)
Alpha ketoglutaric acid.

The list above indicates that other nutrients are needed for
proper B_6 metabolism. The last is a naturally occurring substance in the body. It is part of the body's citric acid, or energy,
cycle. It can be great help for those with fatigue, hypoglycemia
and bladder allergy. Unfortunately, its long name keeps many
from recommending it. Citric acid itself can be supplemented
to help balance the energy cycle. Be careful as this nutrient is
usually derived from (fungal) fermentation and not citrus fruits.
   Finally the body must be able to convert B_6 from the dietary
form, pyridoxine, to the form the body actually uses which is
called *pyridoxal-5-phosphate* or *P5P*. This conversion is called
PHOSPHORYLATION and occurs in the liver. All the work
done in the body by B_6 is done *solely* by the P5P form! The
pyridoxine form does nothing. And if the liver is not functioning
optimally, it will have less capacity to perform this crucial
phosphorylation. Who has trouble phosphorylating B_6? Yes the
E.I. And also those with more well known liver disorders including hepatitis, alcoholism, mono (or CEBV), and also the
aged. Vitamins B_1 and B_2 are also phosphorylated by the liver.
Thiamine (B_1) becomes thiamine pyrophosphate and
Riboflavin (B_2) becomes Riboflavin-5-Phosphate. Other
nutrients may also be converted to active coenzyme form. Inositol becomes myoinositol and pantothenic acid (B_5) becomes

pantothene.

DIFFICULTY IN PHOSPHORYLATING B-VITAMINS
1. Alcoholics
2. Hepatitis Sufferers
3. Aged
4. Allergic Individuals

Fortunately for the Ecologically Ill, and others with liver disease, several vitamin companies make the phosphorylated vitamins available.

Now you may be aware of the B_6 controversy of 1983.[56] The media played up a medical report of six patients who suffered neurological complaints from B_6 megadoses. These had actually been prescribed by M.D.'s and ranged from 1-6 grams! Note that all the symptoms vanished after B_6 was halted. As we have said B_6 can be crucial to the Ecologically Ill, we will list some possible causes for the above neurological complaints. First the dosages are way out of line. Almost never is more than 100-200 milligrams needed. In fact with the P5P form 50 mgs is plenty. It is not true, as some books by medical nutritionists seem to indicate, that more is always better. Pyridoxine belongs to a class of chemicals, pyrimidines, that can be toxic to the nervous system. Also as the FDA allows certain amounts of impurities, this gets magnified with large doses. So allergies or toxicities from excipients is always a possibility. The lack of any B_6 supporting nutrients, listed above, did not allow B_6 to function properly either.

Finally, the science of enzyme kinetics tells us how biochemical reactions take place.[57] A little extra pyridoxine should lead to extra P5P being made, but excess of pyridoxine may *saturate* the system and prevent P5P from being made. And recall that the P5P form is needed for many things—*including* proper neurological functioning! Thus the excess amounts of pyridoxine may have actually caused a *deficiency* of the Pyridoxal-5-Phosphate form which may have been the cause of the symptoms!! In conclusion, taking small amounts of P5P (and the other phosphorylated vitamins) may be very beneficial to the E.I.

Another recent topic in nutrition is *ESSENTIAL FATTY ACID* (**EFA** *OR VIT. F) METABOLISM*.

We will have only a rudimentary discussion here. There are three forms of EFA. All are needed in appropriate amounts. Often the E.I. have deficiencies of the first two (below) and/or excesses of the third. The three EFA's are converted to PROS-TAGLANDINS in the body. These are hormone-like substances secreted by virtually all cells. They were first found in prostate secretions, hence the name. Prostaglandins can regulate or interact with the nervous, circulatory and immune systems. They can benefit or harm these systems as we shall see.

The first EFA we'll look at, is called linoleic acid. It's found in sunflower seeds and linseed oil. After several metabolic steps, the body should convert it to gamma linolenic acid. If it can't, evening primrose oil and black currant oil are the only known food sources for the latter form of this EFA. Finally the gamma linolenic acid is converted to prostaglandin E_1 (also denoted variously as PE_1 or PG_1). To get to PG_1, B_6, zinc, magnesium, Vit. C., and niacin are needed. The second form of EFA is called EPA or eicosapentanoic acid. It's found in salmon, mackerel, sardines and other fish. From EPA, the body makes prostaglandin E_3 or PG_3. Finally the third form of EFA is called arachidonic acid and is found in peanuts and red meats. The body makes this into prostaglandin E_2 or PG_2.

Now the PG_2, in excess, can lead to inflammatory and circulatory disorders. Aspirin works by inhibiting its synthesis. (Aspirin also inhibits Vit. C and interferon syntheses.) *Increasing* PG_1 and PG_3 can inhibit excess PG_2 formation in a natural way. Eskimos eating fish oil containing EPA (despite very high cholesterol content) is how they have virtually no cardiovascular disease! Many people are probably eating too much of the third EFA (from peanuts and red meats) and are deficient in the first two EFA's above. Some nutritionists, though, say that red meat once a week is a good idea. (Some arachidonic acid is necessary.) The first two types of EFA have been touted as benefiting those with arthritis, PMS, MS and other degenerative disorders. Here again is where muscle testing comes in handy. Virtually everyone we tested for sensitivity to evening primrose oil used to test *weak*. We took everyone off of it! It was doing more harm than good. It turned out that hexane was used to extract the nutrients from the plant! Now hexane-free primrose oil is available. But hexane is still often used in "standardized potency" herbal supplements! Remember also that most oils go rancid very easily. The E.I. are very susceptible to the free radicals in rancid oils. Black currant is also available or you can rotate your supplements.

Now we come to one of the final frontiers of nutrition — **AMINO ACID (A.A.) METABOLISM.**
Again we can only have a rudimentary discussion here. Amino acids are the building blocks of all proteins in the body. This includes hormones (like insulin) and neurotransmitters (chemicals that are secreted and absorbed by nerve cells — thus allowing all nerve transmission). This facilitates how we move, think and feel. A.A.'s also are the building blocks of cellular and digestive enzymes, and structural proteins as found in your hair and nails. Philpott has written that amino acid testing is the "window to the body's metabolism."[58] He recommends a 24-hour urine test for amino acids. Urine testing is preferred over blood as the former allows for information on kidney processing. But both can be done. This author co-invented kinesiological testing for amino acids in 1981, but that is beyond our scope here.

We note that vitamins and minerals are cofactors (helpers) in the metabolism of amino acids. The chemist depicts this as follows.

$$A.A._1 \overset{\text{Vit.}}{\underset{\text{Min.}}{\Rightarrow}} A.A._2$$

A.A. will be our abbreviation for amino acid, henceforth. Now vitamins and minerals cannot correct for amino acid deficiencies or improper metabolisms in and of themselves. Supplementing with amino acids and diet changes are what is needed. We're ready now to discuss some individual amino acids.[59]

First, we list the so-called *ESSENTIAL AMINO ACIDS*. They are lysine, tryptophan, leucine, isoleucine, valine, methionine, phenylalanine and threonine. Classically these eight are called essential because the body can (theoretically) make all the others from these eight, but these eight must be present in the diet. Until five years ago, it was thought that all eight must be present in a meal *simultaneously* to facilitate proper protein metabolism (anabolism). This is where the concept of complementary foods came in. Such a combination was beans and grains. The grains are low in lysine. This would then be the *limiting* amino acid. The amount of the latter—the essential A.A. present in the least amount—in a grain meal, would determine how much protein synthesis could take place. This is why beans, high in lysine, would be added to the meal. So all essential A.A. would be present in equivalent amounts. It is now known that such complementing need not occur at the same meal, as blood levels of amino acids remain high for at least 8-12 hours. So complementing can occur for several meals during the day. This is good news for vegetarians, as meats more often have "full" protein (A.A.s) levels than do vegetable foods.

Two A.A.s are said to be *SEMI-ESSENTIAL*. This means during one's lifetime, there are periods when the body can not make sufficient amounts of these A.A.s from the essential A.A.s. The semi-essential A.A.s are thus "essential" at certain times. Histidine is needed in the diet during infancy. And arginine is needed in the diet during the rapid growth years of adolescence. It's incorporated into growth hormone.

The remaining A.A.s are said to be *NON-ESSENTIAL*. These include GABA, glutamic acid, tyrosine, glycine, aspartic acid, citrulline, ornithine, glutamine, cystine, cysteine, taurine, serine. They can be made from the essential ones by the body. But this is for the "theoretically healthy, average person" and does not allow for individuality or Environmental Illness. In fact, many people cannot make several of the "non-essential" A.A.s from the essential A.A.s. Thus the non-essential A.A.s become "essential" to them. They must be supplemented with or added via diet. This is also why some testing for A.A.s is crucial. Never attempt to match symptoms with deficiencies of A.A.s (or other nutrients). Especially if medical or other testing is available.

Let's now look at how some A.A.s become hormones .and neurotransmitters. A neurotransmitter, recall, is the chemical secreted by one nerve cell and absorbed by the next. It quickly moves across the space (synapse) between them. Though our brains are perhaps the most intricate entities known in the universe, its individual connections work simply. A neurotransmitter can do only one of two things. It can increase (excitatory) or decrease (inhibitory) the rate of firing of the next nerve cell that absorbs it.

The amino acid tryptophan is converted into the inhibitory neurotransmitter, serotonin. Vitamins B_3, B_6, C and carbohydrates are needed here. If B_3 (niacin) is low, tryptophan will actually be made into niacin instead of serotonin. Deficiencies of serotonin can cause insomnia, depression, obsessive-compulsive behavior, and sensitivity to bright lights and loud sounds. It's easy to see how the inhibitory nature of serotonin can account for these symptoms. Our brains work to inhibit continuous signals. That's why you may feel the chair you are sitting on when you first sit down. But our brains have better things to do than to be continuously aware of this, so after a few seconds these signals are inhibited and we no longer feel the chair. But if signals are not inhibited, sounds and lights seem intense and emotions may become compulsive. Serotonin is also regulated by negative ions which can thus alleviate some of the symptoms above as well as asthma and sinusitis. Melatonin (readily available now as the sleep hormone) is also made from tryptophan. Its release is triggered by sunlight (through the skull) acting on the pineal.

After several deaths ten years ago, some governments banned tryptophan supplements, though it was still sold in baby formulas and many other ways. The problem was that the Japanese petrochemical giant, Showa Denko made toxic forms of tryptophan. There is nothing inherently wrong with this *essential* amino acid. But 5OH (5-Hydroxy) Tryptophan is now readily available instead of tryptophan. The newer form is actually more potent and is only one metabolic step from serotonin.

Phenylalanine can suppress appetite by its action on the Appestat. With iron as a cofactor, it's made into the A.A. tyrosine. Tyrosine, with iodine, becomes the thyroid hormone, thyroxine. Tyrosine also becomes the neurotransmitter, dopamine. Parkinson's disease is a dopamine disorder. Tyrosine also becomes the well known hormone/neurotransmitter adrenalin (epinephrine) and the lesser known noradrenalin (norepinephrine). Phenylalanine and tyrosine can also become the monoamines phenylethylamine and tyramine respectively. Recall from Chapter 11, that excess levels of monoamines can cause headaches and faulty blood pressure. Bacterial overgrowths can also create toxic levels of these substances.[60]

Histidine is converted into histamine which also acts as a neurotransmitter. Histamine is often either too low (paradoxically) or too high in allergic individuals and schizophrenics. Arthritics are often low in histidine, especially rheumatoid arthritics. Histidine is found in radishes which may be why this family of foods can cause watery eyes, etc. Histidine is also related to sexual functioning. Histidine is low in those who have trouble attaining orgasm, and is high in those who have premature ejaculation. Food for thought? Other factors may be involved here. Muscle testing can tell you if you really want to be with your partner, in case you can't tell!

Glutamine (excitatory) can actually cross the blood-brain barrier and energize the brain almost like glucose. It is used to overcome addictions, overeating and for memory enhancement. Remember, though, never take A.A.s unless tests reveal you need them! Glutamine can be converted to GABA (inhibitory) and to glutamic acid. GABA is often low in Candidiasis patients. The EFA arachidonic acid can also act as a neurotransmitter and choline (a B-Vitamin), becomes the major neurotransmitter, acetylcholine. Disorders with the last substance are involved in Alzheimer's

Disease, which has been linked, along with most other degenerative neurological disorders, to environmental toxins.

Deficiencies of lysine and/or excesses of arginine are involved with Herpes. Arginine is found in chocolate, wheat and other foods. Leucine, isoleucine and valine are so called *branched chain* A.A.s. They are shaped like a "Y". They comprise 30% of muscle mass. Leucine deficiency can also cause improper glucose metabolism. Threonine (often low in the E.I.) is said to be difficult to be absorbed. Texts state that deficiencies are associated with people that are "irritable and difficult to be around."

Let's look at methionine metabolism now. The body ideally makes methionine into cysteine, cystine and taurine successively, in this order. (These A.A.s are all sulfur containing A.A.s. Cysteine, primarily, is incorporated into most structural proteins. If you burn your skin or hair, it will smell of sulfur — like a rotten egg.) We know from Ch. 5, that methionine is often not metabolized properly in the E.I. Instead we've said that toxic, addictive, endorphin-like substances are created. Blood and urine assays look for these. If improperly metabolized, methionine should be avoided. It's found in beans, eggs and "lipotrophic [fat metabolizing] factors" in the health food stores. Cysteine and/or taurine are often deficient in the E.I. Taurine deficiency can cause epilepsy, cardiac arrhythmia, insomnia and excessive jerking while in the act of falling asleep. For eliminating epilepsy: taurine, magnesium, B6 and allergy elimination have been extremely successful as has energy balancing! Taurine and glycine are made into bile. Bile disorders are also common in the E.I.

The kidneys may spill taurine. The peptides (composed of several A.A.s), carnosine and anserine can *shock* the kidneys into *failing to* reabsorb taurine. The kidneys, at one stage filter out most of the blood's components. At a later stage, they will reabsorb a purified version of these components — including A.A.s. Taurine may not be reabsorbed. This syndrome is called "pseudo-allergic reaction" as eating most meats can cause the following symptoms: headaches, fatigue, irritability, and epilepsy. The meats involved include beef, lamb, pork, chicken, duck, turkey, rabbit, salmon and tuna. (Note the last two are America's most popular and canned fish; perhaps we could call this pseudo-allergy/addiction syndrome.) Don't overeat meats; if tests reveal this syndrome, elimination of most meats together with amino acid supplementation has been employed. This factor along with the arachidonic acid content may be why some feel better when they cut back or eliminate red meat.

Did you know that the body makes *AMMONIA*? Does your urine or menstrual flow ever smell like ammonia? Are you very sensitive to it? The liver's urea cycle helps rid the body of ammonia. Excess ammonia can damage the nerve sheaths. It can also cause confusion, headaches, inability to concentrate and food allergies.[61] Philpott has found that a few cases of ALS (Amyotrophic Lateral Sclerosis or Lou Gehrig's disease) were helped by eliminating excess ammonia accumulations.[62] (Low protein and an allergy-free diet would be used.) Threonine has recently become the preferential amino acid to help clear ammonia from the body and brain. (Glutamic acid and aspartic acid may have previously been used for this purpose but may no longer be recommended.)

Glutamic acid is also used as a stomach acid supplement in some digestive enzymes. It may be preferable to the usual betaine hydrochloride — a beet derivative. Aspartic acid is a precursor of nucleic acids which make up our genetic material — RNA and DNA.

Carnitine helps transport fatty acids across our cells' energy factories — the mitochondria. After a heart attack, carnitine levels, in the heart, often drop to zero, making it crucial for the sufferer. Such information is found by M.D.'s and then ignored, by other (orthodox) M.D.'s, as amino acids can't be patented. Glutathione is a tri-peptide and powerful anti-oxidant, as we have stated. Along with Vit. C and taurine, it's being found useful for cataracts. Purchase "reduced glutathione" only. Arginine and ornithine are incorporated into thymic and growth hormones. The latter also is a fat metabolizer. As such, they have been touted in weight reduction supplements. But they are often improperly metabolized — so be careful. Glycine (inhibitory) is found in the spinal cord and is a bile constituent. It's also needed for proper glucose metabolism and hemoglobin formation.

Never take excess A.A.s or untested A.A.s as they may stress the kidneys and other organs. And never take "full spectrum" A.A. supplements as many people have improper metabolism of one or more A.A.s. But do get tested (with blood/urine or kinesiology) for amino acid metabolism. (See Appendix B.) Correcting deficiencies and improper metabolisms can be crucial to getting well.

A final note on "21st Century" nutrition. With advanced kinesiological methods, underlying factors behind a nutritional deficiency *can* be identified *and* balanced, in priority fashion, analogous to the Candida Balance. There are reasons why some never seem to need supplementation and others who consume megadoses never overcome their symptoms.[63]

In more detail, if MBT indicates a nutritional deficiency, advanced procedures let the body reveal if other imbalances (meridian, emotional, structural, etc.) are the cause. Half the time, factors — other than nutritional — are revealed for nutritional deficiencies! Then these other factors can be balanced or corrected. So we see that most nutrition, as currently practiced, is in the dark ages.

Here in the fourth edition, we are pleased to report on a new nutrient — Microhydrin™. This is a patented anti-oxidant comprised of silica hydride. Its ionized hydrogen is 1000 times more potent an anti-oxidant than Vitamin C! More importantly, our research has revealed that in many people, it can prevent some reactions to foods if taken beforehand or it can halt some reactions even after they have begun if one has eaten something one is reacting to. Unlike the touted MSM, this supplement actually can halt gastrointestinal permeability. Please contact us about obtaining Microhydrin.™

14

SCIENCE, MEDICINE AND SOCIETY

In this chapter, we will have a no-holds-barred discussion on whether MBT is scientific and on whether western medicine is scientific. We will show that the arguments used by the medical orthodoxy against alternative healing modalities are, in fact, not arguments of scientific logic. And that the medical physician is not a scientist and usually does not know what science is. We will highlight this with numerous examples of medical nightmares of this century (some of which are still going on) all under the false guise of science. We will see that the epidemic ills of society will force the acceptance of our two-model approach to wellness.

First, we will demonstrate that western medicine is ignorant of scientific reasoning much of the time. As a physicist, this is an easy task to demonstrate. The three major arguments used by orthodox physicians are as follows.[64] (1) To be scientific, one must know how or why a healing method—like MBT—works. (2) To be scientific, one must understand a healing method—like MBT—at the microscopic level. A macroscopic (large or human-level) understanding is insufficient. (3) Double-blind, statistical studies are both necessary and sufficient to prove scientific validity.

The first argument demonstrates that medicine does not comprehend what science is all about. We will use the phenomenon of gravity to show this. Some 300 years ago, Isaac Newton was supposedly hit on the head by a falling apple. He deduced that the same force pulls all objects at the Earth's surface to its core and also holds the solar system together. He even described this force in terms of masses and distances. But did Newton know *why* masses attract with the forces they exhibit? Do physicists *now* know why? The answer both times is categorically *no!* Only recently with remarkably complex theories of quantum, relativistic gravity called superstring theory, are physicists making some inroads into the why of gravity. But have physicists dismissed gravity as "anecdotal?" Of course not. Men travelled to the moon, and baseballs are made all with the "anecdotal" knowledge of gravity.

And this century's discovery of quantum physics led to the Copenhagen Interpretation which specifically stated that if a theory works conclusively, that's all that matters at the moment. Experimental verification takes precedence over whether or not the theorists know "why." Indeed, all that a "law" of nature is, is the simple consistent observation that condition A leads to condition B. How or why is not a prerequisite to having a "law" of nature. Thus we do not need to know how or why, precisely, MBT works at the moment, if its consistent benefits are proven. And whoever gives it a chance invariably sees the consistent benefits. Meteorologists make the same mistake physicians do. They won't accept the farmer's findings on how animal behavior can predict the weather months ahead of time. Everything must come from computer models of "known" variables. As a consequence, the farmer's almanac often offers a more accurate forecast, months ahead of time, than the weatherman does for the next day!

Now for #2. An observation or understanding at the microscopic level is not a necessity or correct argument of science either. The author's doctoral advisor in Physics, Professor Max Dresden, wrote a paper called, "Reflections on Fundamentality and Complexity."[65] He cited several phenomenon which could be understood at either microscopic or macroscopic levels. These include temperature and turbulence. At the microscopic level, the laws of particle interactions yield the observed results. But macroscopic variables like air pressure also yield the same results. Therefore, though the scales are related, either scale is sufficient by itself to have a scientific understanding of a phenomenon.[66] In ecological matters, if a person becomes arthritic after eating wheat, you don't need to see his joint cells "sneeze" from the allergic reaction. It is proven at the macroscopic or "human" level! And how MBT works at the cellular level is not needed at the moment either. We note that many drugs and surgical procedures are, in fact, exempted by physicians from their own incorrect arguments. These specious arguments are often reserved to fool the media and the people (in a self-serving way) against new or alternative treatments.

Finally, let's look at argument #3. Double-blind, statistical studies are not needed to demonstrate scientific validity. Studies on the solar system have never been done with and without the planets. As a bona fide scientist, I have been shocked when reading the medical, "scientific" literature. I can recall reading an issue of the leading American medical (trade) publication. Most of the articles pertained to drugs. About half were proclaiming that double-blind, statistical, "scientific" studies just proved the safety and efficacy of a new wonder drug. But the other half of these articles were warnings that new studies revealed that last year's or the last decade's new wonder drug was neither safe nor efficient! But these drugs too had been "proven" by double-blind, statistical studies! So how *scientific* could medicine's mythical, double-blind, statistical studies be?! Of course, more and more, it is being revealed that medical researchers and physicians often "doctor" the experiments to get the results they want.

Upon entering the health field, a decade ago, this physicist was shocked to see that the results of a study could be predicted based upon *who paid for the study*. If the dairy industry provides the "research" grant, milk and cheese will always be found to have great health benefits and no possible harm — in contradistinction to reality. And it is indeed easy to doctor a statistical study. In a graduate mathematics course, the professor told us the standard joke that there are three kinds of lies: little lies, big lies and *statistics*. Regarding the drug industry, such studies often are a cover-up to support the masking of symptoms with foreign, toxic substances when usually there is a much better and safer, natural remedy available.

Indeed the very premise of modern medicine – that of matching a drug for each symptom is the very epitome of pseudo-science and ultimately of anti-science. *Whenever possible,* science deals with cause and effect. Can the cause of a symptom possibly be "drug deficiency?" Pharmacological studies are thus irrelevant to the issue of whether drug use is scientific *in the first place*. Of course, there are many modern, medical triumphs which have utilized science and technology, such as the microsurgical reattachment of limbs. But for most chronic, degenerative, physical, emotional and immunological disease; the impotence of modern medicine belies its lack of scientific validity!

Now we are saddened to see some "holistic" physicians denigrate MBT too. For some, this indicates that they are not yet holistic. More physicians are turning to nutrition and this is a good and necessary step. But they often think, as do their more orthodox colleagues, that health can only come from popping a pill or receiving an intravenous (vitamin) injection. They have thus made only an infinitesimal paradigm shift in their thinking. Many of these physicians may need the MACHINE to interface with their patients. Allergy testing can only be done via needles, blood taking or new electric devices. They don't seem to want to be with their patients or touch them for an hour. (Fortunately, many truly holistic physicians, like the one that wrote this book's foreword, enjoy balancing and touching their patients.)

MBT is denounced, by some in the alternative field, as "subjective." Well, quantum physics proved that all testing is subjective and will alter that which it is testing! The above methods are notoriously inaccurate for food allergy *and* sensitivity testing. And all blood work entails its own inaccuracies. When I was ill, over 25% of my (many) blood tests were either lost or had improbable results! The truth is that MBT, if used properly, can, by its very low energy-sensing nature, detect sensitivities and imbalance *not detectable* in any other way at present.

One of the real enemies of the people, in this matter, are the orthodox allergists. When the media or their medical colleagues ask them if schizophrenia or arthritis can be caused by food or chemical allergy, or if systemic Candidiasis exists, they yell, "NO." They are content to "treat" hay fever, hives, asthma, and rashes with their perennial allergy injections. Food and chemical allergies are often totally ignored in favor of "treatable" pollen allergy. This is a crime against the people, as anyone with pollen allergies usually has food and chemical allergies affecting them a thousand times more! Dr. Mendlesohn showed that allergy injections often don't work and can even be fatal — see Ref. 11. (Sometimes the symptoms change to the systemic kind that are unrecognized by the allergists.)

The media is also a key enemy of the people here. This is in connection with Federal agencies such as the FDA and the FCC. Ineffective, over-the-counter drugs can have television commercials aired, but nutritional and other natural remedies are not allowed the same right. When a new alternative method becomes known, the "Health and Science" reporter interviews one of a handful of (self-appointed "expert") M.D.'s about it. He invariably states that the method is "untried, unscientific, not beneficial and likely very harmful." This is in spite of the facts that he knows *nothing* about the alternative method, wouldn't know what science is if it hit him in the face, and the usual medical treatment for this ill is *in fact* ineffective and known to be harmful! Why does the media act this way? Just wait for the commercial after the "Health and Science" report. Yes, it's a drug ad!

Large foundations for cancer, arthritis, gastrointestinal illness and many other degenerative ills cry "fraud" when diet is said to be the cause. Yet the facts are many of these ills, like cancer and cardiovascular disease, didn't even exist until this century when the food, air and water were altered. Most arthritic specialists, gastroenterologists, dermatologists, and psychiatrists would be out of a job if the ecological model were used. And if prevention were added, most cancer specialists, diabetologists and cardiovascular specialists would also be looking for jobs. Most doctor visits are for fatigue. These would be obviated too if the energy and ecology models were employed. Likewise many doctor visits are iatrogenic — doctor caused — in the first place. The human and financial costs here could easily be obviated if MBT were routinely used. MBT is a dream come true — a method virtually *free of side effects* yet capable of true healing! All this points to the fact that if the two-model approach of this book were used, the savings to society could approach a *trillion* dollars a year, in the U.S. alone! People were meant to have up to about a hundred years of good health and then die in their sleep. And we can all have this, if we assume the responsibility for our health.

Addiction to drugs like cocaine, heroine, and alcohol are tearing our society apart. But why are these addictions rampant *today*? These substances have been available for hundreds and thousands of years. It is precisely because we have become an addicted society. As foods, chemicals, etc. affect mood so readily, addictions result. The medical model supports taking alien substances to alter moods. So if one is "down" often, say from an (unknowing) food allergy withdrawal, using "recreational" drugs is a "logical" next step in our society. To end this vicious cycle of addiction, education is a key element. Preventing sugar or wheat addiction is part of preventing cocaine and alcohol addiction. And if society demands drug-urine screening, what about the pilot or train conductor who is "out of it" because he's high on milk or chocolate.

And once you know the ecology model, it is clear how many national leaders have suffered from the HAC Syndrome. Regardless of the -ism, whether a Brezhnev or a Nixon, the kind of person often driven to power-cravings is often the last person who should have it. Hypoglycemia with its accompanying hyperadrenalism (which results in emotional imbalance, and sometimes great drive) was a likely factor in Nixon and even Hitler. The excess weight of a Brezhnev or of mass-killers like the "Son of Sam" and the hospital nurse on Long Island point to allergy-addiction. The Son of Sam is known to have many food cravings, the nurse suffered from depression. Hitler was known to have colitis and severe cigarette allergy. (Anyone who smoked near him was likely to soon be hanging by piano wire.) How many millions have lost their lives because imbalanced, ecologically ill and power crazy men have ruled? The psychiatrists may write their little books about these rulers' mental ills, but the ecology model is much more relevant and accurate. So we see that society suffers in ways we may not have imagined.

The collusion between the medical, pharmaceutical and food processing industries must be exposed and countered.[67] In school, we are all taught to eat from the "four food groups everyday." This is precisely what starts an allergy-addiction cycle. Instead the fact that any physical and emotional complaint can arise from what you eat, drink or breathe should be taught in the public schools. Along with the recommendation to *not* eat the same foods everyday and the recognition of addictions.

We envision that every family will one day know how to do their own MBT precluding much addiction, illness and doctor visits. If the energy and ecology balancing models are taught to all, we can again have a happy, healthy society. After all, how many people do you know that don't have headaches, arthritis, fatigue, stomach aches, high or low blood pressure, high or low blood sugar, learning problems, poor memory and balance, emotional disorders, skin problems, and other chronic problems? With the non-medical testing and balancing methods in this book, every family can learn how to get and keep themselves well! After all, MBT and balancing is virtually devoid of possible harm and has the limitless potential for wellness.

To further prove our point, that orthodox medicine's claim to be scientific is literally obscene, we will cite several examples of medical treatments in this century— some are still going on. What these examples demonstrate is that the Western physician at any time acts as if he possesses *all knowledge and ultimate knowledge*. Both claims are absurd and unscientific.

TWENTIETH CENTURY MEDICAL " SCIENCE"

#1. Because the thymus gland shrank when a person was ill, it was removed up to the 1950's when it was discovered to *merely* be the master gland of the immune system!

#2. Minor skin (e.g. acne or pimples) and thyroid problems (both undoubtedly due to energy and ecology imbalance) were routinely treated with X-rays and other radiation! Some of this may still be going on! The result has been death, cancer, or a life-time of drug dependency (as a result, e.g., of a destroyed thyroid).

#3. Since fiber in food could not be digested and had "no nutrients," it could be removed from food. Here is a link between the medical and food processing industries. Resulting low fiber diets have been proven to cause cancer, cardiovascular and gastrointestinal disease. Again the Western physician here assumed his knowledge and wisdom were greater than that of nature. Or was it the food industry's desire for long-term, cheap food storage? Bugs don't eat food without fiber—they know where the nutrients are!

#4. Pediatricians have recommended mothers use "formula" (note the scientific sounding name) instead of nature's own blessing— breast milk. Countless millions now have weak immune systems because of this! Numerous vitamins, minerals, amino acids and other food components are not found in cow's milk or other contrived, mass-produced "formulas." Mother's milk also contains antibodies to strengthen the baby's immune system. Here, under the false guise of science, pediatricians pretended to have all and ultimate knowledge and thus committed this medical blasphemy against nature. Even using artificial nipples has been shown to lead to dental and TMJ (jaw) defects, and what about the loss of bonding? Pediatricians today say, "mother's milk is better, but formula is just as good"?! At every age, western physicians, if they ever do admit a mistake, will try to seduce you into believing that the new formula, or the new drug or the new artificial sweetener is now O.K. But you know what will happen in 10 years.

#5. Cancer is due to viruses and should only be treated by drugs, radiation and surgery. The facts are that after spending over $20 billion since the 1970 "war on cancer," the 300,000 yearly death rate has reached 500,000 now! M.D.'s, drug companies and "researchers" (looking for the viruses, e.g.) have gotten rich at the expense of the lives of millions. Let's look at a comparison between physics and medicine. With the freedom of the world at stake, the U.S. government declared a "war" on the atom in 1942. Some two billion dollars was spent on the Manhattan Project for nuclear scientists and metallurgists to come up with a new "Atom Bomb". Within about two years, the goal was achieved. But in medicine after decades and ten times the funding, medical people have not achieved their goal. The answer, as indicated above, is clear. The entire premise is unsound and unscientific. Looking for (toxic) pills as the "cure" for a disease caused by other toxins is really quite absurd. In fact, most chemotherapies and radiation are known to cause cancer!

As cancer hardly existed at the turn of the century, the ecological causation is clearly indicated. The three "approved" anti-cancer methods all *destroy* an already weak immune system. Is it any wonder they don't work? Putting more poison in an already poisoned system is anything but science! Since the 1920's, some leading medical doctors have had various effective, natural anti-cancer remedies. They have always been persecuted and prosecuted. Their research is rejected from the medical journals they're submitted to. Then, in typical medical double-talk, the orthodoxy cries, "show me the literature, show me the studies." Fifty years after Dr. Gerson employed vegetables and their juices in his cancer therapy (and was persecuted), the orthodoxy *now* admits various vitamins contained in these vegetables *do* help prevent cancer. The truth is cancer can readily be prevented and if any of the natural treatments available were first employed (instead of being a last ditch effort, as is usually the case after conventional therapies destroy the immune system) most could be saved. In this country, spineless lawmakers are bought by the medical lobbies, making it illegal to treat cancer in natural ways. So much for freedom in western countries. If you don't have the freedom to save your life, how much are the other freedoms worth? The growing number of medical physicians who treat cancer with natural means—jeopardizing their licenses— are to be highly commended.

#6. The surgical removal of the breasts of 12 year-old girls because their mothers and grandmothers had breast cancer. This may still occur in some parts of the U.S. and the world! Here the medical fondness for statistical studies reaches maddening proportions. The ignorance of underlying ecological factors in favor of a *statistical* understanding is the "logic" here. What the evidence really indicates is that the young girl should be taught that if she doesn't dye her hair, avoids caffeine, cigarettes and similar substances, and takes Vitamins E and B6, she can likely avoid what is only a genetic *predisposition to ecological imbalance!*

#7. The large arthritis industry vehemently denies that diet is a cause of arthritis. Instead drugs can be the only answer. Here the folly is that most arthritics become allergic to the very toxic drugs used. This could only be expected as the arthritic is a very allergic person and ingesting something everyday, we saw, leads to allergy! As with cancer and most medical epidemics today, politics and economics, and not lives and true science, are what count to the medical orthodoxy.

#8. The recommendation to take an aspirin or two a day to prevent cardiovascular disease based on "scientific studies." Aspirin is, in fact, a highly allergenic (salicylate) compound. It can cause ulcers and Reye's Syndrome. The latter can result in severe illness and death in children who take aspirin while they have the flu or chicken pox. Here is another example of medical double-talk. Many nutrients (see Ch. 11) work better than aspirin to prevent cardiovascular ills and without possible side-effects. Thus we see the paranoid medical views of vitamin-as-drug and drug-as vitamin?!

#9. The myths of dietary cholesterol and salt as causing cardiovascular disease (CVD) and high blood pressure respectively. Though blood vessel diseases are associated with cholesterol buildup, the ingestion of foods containing cholesterol is not the cause. The body makes far more cholesterol than is found in most peoples' diets. (Cholesterol is needed to coat the blood vessels to facilitate blood flow.) Eskimos are free of CVD even though they do eat foods (fish blubber) higher in cholesterol than many people with CVD who had low-cholesterol diets. And allergies, nutritional deficiencies and metabolic disorders (of B_6 and the amino acid cysteine) have been proven to cause CVD. Likewise, the chapter on heart integration listed foods that can cause high blood pressure. Avoiding these foods and all allergens and performing the Rochlitz Heart Integration exercise will normalize blood pressure even if a high salt diet is maintained. Nations with diets high in salt but low in dairy products usually have populations with a low incidence of high blood pressure, again proving this point. The medical profession apparently can't discern association from causation. Something scientists are trained to do.

#10. Studies in several countries (the first one being Israel) revealed that when doctors went on strike, the death rate invariably went down! The lesson is self-explanatory.

#11. The repeated brazen attempts to outlaw dietary and nutritional counseling except that from M.D.'s. While, of course, the vast majority of M.D.'s have never taken a nutrition course!

#12. "It's Genetic." This is another catch-all phrase that the medical orthodoxy uses when they don't know much about an illness. It, like "stress", can be used to "explain" away anything. Of course the truth is almost always that a dietary or ecological factor is really the relevant cause. Many "genetic" ills are really a genetic predisposition to an intolerance to certain foods. Knowing this, a "genetic" illness may easily be obviated through diet changes, etc.

#13. Newborns and young infants, until just the last couple of years, were said to have an incomplete nervous system. Therefore, they probably did not feel pain until some (arbitrary) later age. So they could be operated on without any anesthesia!! Maybe all the screams have caused the present awareness by the medical orthodoxy. They now "scientifically" realize that newborns feel pain!! We think there may be a more insidious factor. Perhaps there were no safe anesthetics (until recently) that would render the young infant unconscious without killing him. So the medical establishment just declared that infants don't need anesthesia. This is, at present, a hypothesis.

#14. The medical orthodoxy often will first look for viruses as the cause of not-yet-understood diseases. Countless billions of dollars spent on scientific-looking research is wasted because (less expensive) diet and ecological factors are not first examined. In reality, the huge industry of medical, microscopic research has its own economic momentum with little actual payoff; because it's not scientifically valid.

#15. Western medicine is quick to give every malady a com-

plex-sounding name. While usually having little or no understanding of the malady. It's an interesting linguistic game they
play at the expense of their patients' health. Patients are brainwashed to feel relieved when the "doctor" tells them the name
of their affliction. But, oftentimes, the name is nothing other
than the Latin translation of their complaint! In fact, this is part
of the problem with the ecologically ill. The medical orthodoxy
doesn't have the names to give these people. The official word
hasn't come down from *Big Medical Brother*. They won't accept
outsider's new names. Candidiasis, kinesiology, Universal Allergies, etc. are not (yet) accepted in Big Medical Brother's
Dictionary. So they don't want their patients to have the relief
afforded by these new names. The orthodoxy realizes if patients
were able to get "name relief" from holistic medical doctors,
chiropractors, naturopaths, kinesiologists, etc., they could lose
their monopoly on name relief. Instead — when they can't come
up with a good medical name — the vague names are used.
These include: "it's genetic", "it's stress", or "it must be
psychological".

#16. "Placebo" research. Medical double-blind, statistical,
studies often involve the use of a placebo. This is supposed to
be a totally inert substance. In the past, this has been an artifi-
cially colored, sugar pill. But most people test allergic to either
or both of these ingredients! So all these medical and
psychological studies are worthless. Now when alternative
(non-drug) methods help patients, the orthodoxy is quick to cry
"placebo effect". In fact, it is easy to prove that the placebo
effect must be responsible for the apparent success of many
(non-fudged) drug studies. We say this because so often a few
years down the road evidence becomes available that the drug
is neither safe nor effective. So how could it have appeared to
work in the first place? One answer is the placebo effect. Here
the gullible, desperately believing in the doctor's magic pill as
cure, were "helped" by their own minds' tricks!

There are many more examples that demonstrate that in this

century, orthodox, Western medical doctors have used methods that were pseudo-scientific, anti-scientific, and harmful to the people and with great regularity. All the while they proclaim themselves as "medical scientists" and declare whatever treatments they choose to make "standard" are "scientific." The law has been usurped, as "standard" treatments, even if truly unscientific and harmful, cannot have legal suits brought against them! The medical lobbyists have placed the lawmakers in their pockets during this century.

This author will always remember the way his doctoral advisor in Physics, Prof. Max Dresden, an internationally distinguished theoretical physicist, denounced the "totality" of the medical profession as unscientific. He knew — as has been written up by famed medical heretic, Robert Mendelsohn, M.D. — that throughout medical school, the exams are almost exclusively simple multiple choice tests. Those who fail can usually repeat courses too. Prof. Dresden apparently granted only an appropriate amount of respect for the medical profession!

I am sure, however, that he would now be impressed with the new breed of truly holistic physicians — like John Wright — and with their *results*. Prof. Dresden came to his conclusion about current medical practice because his life-long health problems went uncorrected. I later showed him evidence that they were allergy-induced. Having taught physics to pre-med students at a major University, I regret not emphasizing conceptualization more and memorizing less.

When I became disastrously ill, I had first hand knowledge that there was little science in current medicine. My horrifying experiences, and those of the thousands of people I have interviewed around the world since then, have led me to the following conclusion. To paraphrase Churchill, never have so few earned so much (fame and fortune) from so many while knowing so *little* about what they are supposed to know — how to get people well! (The true, holistic physician, we have found, would actually be the strongest supporter of this view.) All the while, for the obvious economic and political reasons, effective knowledge known for thousands of years is being hidden and declared "unscientific." We refer to ecology balancing — known at least for 2500 years to the ancient Greeks and energy balancing — known for perhaps 5000 years to the Chinese. And performing one without the other will also be shown to be unscientific.

Yes, we have high praise for some clinical ecologists who risk the wrath of their colleagues for declaring the obvious — that most illness is caused by harmful substances getting into the body. Yet we have seen some clinical ecologists denounce MBT, acupuncture meridian balancing, chiropractic and even nutrition. Some clinical ecologists have been known to say, "I've given you a rotation diet, Nystatin, supplements, vitamin I.V.'s, desensitization treatment and if you're not well, *nothing else* can be done — avoid the 20th Century and live (or die) with this disease." This is what I and many others around the world have been told. But the above quote is just as harmful and *erroneous* as when the orthodox oncologist says to his cancer patient, "I've given you the best radiation and chemotherapy treatments available, I am sorry but *nothing else* can be done; you have three months to live."

We beseech the clinical ecologists to add the methods and ideas of this book to their practices; either by learning these methods themselves or by hiring (or referring to) a well-trained kinesiologist. I, and by now, perhaps 100,000 people have been helped more in a matter of minutes (by the energy balancing) than I, or they, were with several years of "standard" clinical ecology methodology. We know that our forthrightness will not stop leading, open-minded ecologists from recommending this book to their patients. *Regardless*, as a scientist, this author is compelled to state the truth as he sees it.

We also feel the need to inform the reader of the state of affairs awaiting him or her in the world of holistic health or medicine. Quite a few "holistic" M.D.'s are anything but. Their only modality is still the pill and the I.V. (intravenous injection). They often denounce other modalities they don't use just like their orthodox brethren. No knowledge of the body's electrical nature is afforded by them. Some write simplistic articles and books claiming to cure allergies, Candidiasis, Epstein-Barr Virus, etc. with the ole magic pill— an anti-fungal drug or vitamin, etc. Many see their patients again and again without really helping them. They have no way of testing their patients for allergy to vitamins, weight loss powders, etc. that they often sell themselves.

We strongly advise the reader not to see any physician, practitioner, or "expert"—"holistic" or otherwise—for more than 1-3 visits if they do not experience long term relief or cure. What we have is the opposite of the ancient Chinese system. This system provided for payment if, *and only if*, the patient got well. You could get rich if you really could help people. We don't object to that. Often "holistic" physicians—medical nutritionists and ecologists—become quite wealthy because they see their patients so many times without really helping them appreciably. This is a travesty. Often the patient returns again and again because the physician was the first to provide (holistic) name relief. Frequently, little else is gained after many visits.

The only physicians who have great success with allergies, Candida, or Epstein-Barr are the ones with a very eclectic practice. They usually don't write the books or articles claiming simplistic cures. They're too busy taking seminars and learning new things. They include some form of energy balancing in their practice. This is only a very small portion of the *already* small portion of "holistic" physicians and practitioners! This is another reason why the reader has little choice but to become the expert and the "balancer". We've been saddened on numerous occasions when holistic M.D.'s (overseas) take our seminars and are fascinated when they themselves take the blood pressures of other students and see how the heart integration exercise normalizes blood pressure. Then they go back to their practice and forget about it! Somehow it doesn't fit in with the rest of their practice or they're afraid to employ it or even try. Again we say, rely on yourself, you have no choice. Don't look for any excuses. You'll *appear* to find them. And the reader should learn that the fancy "doctor's office" is sometimes paid for with innumerable and unsuccessful patient visits! No, we are not nihilistic (against everything), but we have talked to thousands of people who have become penniless after believing the "experts" would cure their Allergies, Candidiasis, Epstein-Barr, etc.

Consider finding an expert kinesiologist (at least as adjunct) whose office may not have all the (meaningless) trimmings! Become a responsible non-patient. Don't accept the brainwashing that you must avoid the 20th Century to be well. The author never accepted this and that's why he went on to be well. As for our clients, we only accept those who are willing to perform the corrections from this book. As the epilogue indicates, wellness can now be at your very own fingertips.

But we also want the people to know that there are many ignorant and unscrupulous kinesiologists out there too. Avoid any who proclaim "permanent cures" or cures that "work on everyone" or "97.2% of the people." Kinesiologists must make use of the advances made by clinical ecologists in the areas of allergy, Candidiasis, etc. Otherwise energy balancing may be very short-lived. When employed together, energy and ecology balancing become an *intertwined* and true healing science.

What does the future hold? We may be guardedly optimistic as society can no longer tolerate the self-serving orthodox, medical-pharmaceutical complex. The people are beginning to awaken. Their untreated ills are *forcing* them to. More people realize that drugs should be the last, and not the first, avenue to embark upon. The orthodoxy might attempt to label the ideas and methods of this book as alternative, weird, or dangerous. But the truth is that using substances toxic to the body as the *first* approach to disease is *new, alternative and dangerous*! This alternative approach is only 70 years old! Its long term effects have been to place society on the brink of disaster. Due to ecology and energy imbalance, people can't think, understand, work, feel, and love the way human beings were meant to. Drugs can't correct this. Divorce, drug addiction and crime are rampant. Society and the workplace seem to be mirrored in the postal and parcel service here in the U.S.—you can't mail a letter or package without great trepidation, because so many seem to be unwell and unable to function optimally. How many in government and private industry, in managerial positions, make poor decisions that are so costly to society? We intend to get these ideas into the main stream business world shortly. Taking a time management (memory improvement, or speed reading) seminar is worthless, if the executive is suffering from brain fatigue (and energy imbalance) from coffee, sugar, wheat, etc. We might even extrapolate such allergy/addiction to an entire society. In the West, wheat is the main staple and in the East, rice is the primary grain. Perhaps the greater materialistic and even war-like tendencies in the West may, in part, be due to such allergy/addiction?

If society is to be saved from the potential devastation of its own creation, these new (really old) ideas must be adopted. They will be. Even in Physics, it took 20 years for Einstein's conceptualizations to be adopted. Many older physicists had to literally die first! A similar thing will occur in medicine. As over half the country's population take vitamins (despite their physicians' negativity), the new crop of physicians will soon reflect this tendency. And many of these young people will find that nutrition alone won't correct all their ills. Acupuncture meridians, the spine and other "energy systems" must also be balanced to maintain wellness.

We envision a world where, from birth, a person's potential allergy to food and environment is continually monitored. In China, non-medical "foot doctors" have been the first line of "health defense." With the breakthrough of MBT, both energy and ecology can be monitored and the "foot doctors" can and *should be* the family itself! Balance will then be restored to the individual, the family and to society as a whole! There may be self-serving, reactionary measures, but these changes are inevitable!

15

ON "PSYCHOLOGY" & HOW TO BALANCE YOUR EMOTIONS

Now we will follow up on the ideas of the last chapter and demonstrate that psychiatry is the very epitome of the pseudo- and anti-scientific practices of orthodox, western medicine. We will show that this century's accepted and self-proclaimed "scientific" treatments offered by western psychiatrists are in fact *nightmares* of unproven, dangerous and ineffective methodologies. We will reach the conclusion that it is wise to *terminate* this pseudo-specialty now. For there are many non-medical counselors (including kinesiologists) that can provide talk (and other) therapy without the risk of dangerous drugs and other horrendous treatments. This chapter is terribly relevant as all too many with E.I. never see the appropriate practitioner. They just get shuffled through the psychiatric mill. And if the problem is biochemical, then ecological and energy balancing can always come to the rescue. But because we *do* realize that wellness can only be attained if one's emotions are in balance, we will offer several remarkable emotional de-stressing methods from the ranks of MBT.

First we note that the terms "psychology" and "psychiatry" are misnomers in the way they are usually used. They come from the word "psyche" which refers to a non-physical entity. But if we are physical beings and our behavior is governed by a physical entity, the brain, a non-physical entity cannot be the driving force. *By definition*, a non-physical entity *cannot* interact with a physical entity. What can be observed and thus scientifically treated is either overt human behavior or neurobiological studies. The better universities recognize this and do not have "psychology" departments. Rather they have "behavioral sciences" departments and neurobiology departments. One of the hallmarks of science is to *only* talk about that which you can measure in some way. "Psyches" are unmeasurable and probably undefinable! And this is not just semantics. Many in the"psychiatric" profession are adverse to the ecological and energy models precisely because they are ultimately *"psyche-atrists"* and do not fully realize what a science of behavior is about.

TREATMENTS OF 20TH CENTURY PSYCHIATRIC "SCIENCE"

We will demonstrate that they are unscientific, and very dangerous, while ignoring underlying ecological, nutritional and energy causations.

#1. Insulin shock. This method was widely used until the 1940's or so. Here insulin was injected in psychiatric patients to produce a shock that would snap them out of depression, anti-social behavior, etc. (See the movie *FRANCES* to see how this actress' political views were treated by this and other barbaric methods.) The severe low blood sugar induced did indeed shock the brain and the body with such disastrous consequences to life and health that it was discontinued. Of course, while it was used, it was declared "scientific."

#2. The "new, improved" form of shock therapy is electric shock, a.k.a. electroconvulsive therapy (ECT). This is today declared "scientific" and the "best way" to treat recalcitrant, depressive patients. This brilliant idea came from the association that epileptics have little or no known depression. So why not induce an electrical (epileptic) seizure? Though there may be phony studies that appear to support this, they are anything but scientifically written and performed. Here again we see that the physician acts as frustrated physicist or chemist. While their medical colleagues employ the physicist's devices to treat physical ills — like the use of x-rays and ultraviolet radiation to treat pimples and acne — the psychiatrist wants to play physicist with a complex, fragile electrochemical entity, he knows very little about — the brain! First, this method ignores the scientifically proven research that depression is caused by allergies and nutritional deficiencies and can be easily corrected with methods that deal with these causes.

Then, of course, there is the fact that the treatment is worse than the disease! We will show that this is true of *all* standard psychiatric treatments!! Side-effects of ECT are memory loss and zombie-like behavior. (Of course, each year, it is proclaimed, "the new, improved" ECT voltage won't do this anymore.) One example is the great American novelist, Ernest Hemingway. He is said to have killed himself "out of depression." What really happened is that he allowed himself to be subjected to ECT for his depression. With the resultant memory loss, he was incapable of writing anymore and therefore took his own life. Why did he have depression in the first place? We can only guess, but his heavy drinking and overweight condition are give-aways. These are signs of the HAC syndrome. Randolph showed in the 30's and 40's that the withdrawal from allergies (and alcoholic beverages) leads to a depressive state. Alcohol also induces nutritional deficiencies associated with depression. Through ecological, nutritional and energy balancing modalities, Hemingway could easily have cured his depression. Likewise for the millions of others who suffer from hypothetical "psychiatric" disorders.

#3. Schizophrenia. Here the psychiatrists have never even been able to come up with a consistent definition! Absurd mental models and chemical treatments have never worked. Among the first works on the subject were lists of definitive symptoms made during institutional observations. These included the patient's saying that the "food was poisoning" him and that he could smell the gas stove hundreds of feet away! Yes, the mental institution was the first home-away-from-home for the E.I.!! Some psychiatrists have gone beyond the standard ideas here and have embraced clinical ecology. The psychiatric journals have even allowed the publication of articles linking wheat and milk allergy to schizophrenia. (We like to say that 10% of psychiatrists accept the link of schizophrenia to wheat and milk allergy and the other 90% eat wheat and milk.)

#4. The intellectual "seduction," as Prof. Dresden used to call it, of the Western Medical Establishment by the pseudo-scientific ideas of Sigmund Freud and his followers in the "psychoanalytical" movement. Here, the unproven theories and treatments of Freud, Jung and the neo-Freudians were adopted very readily *in the U.S.*, preferentially. Why? We can guess. If you have to see your analyst one or more times, a week, for five years to get better, you can certainly enrich him and your fantasies simultaneously. The book, *THE PSYCHOLOGICAL SOCIETY*, by Martin L. Gross demonstrates that all the analysts' theories on the unconscious are nonsense.[68] The one thing missing there is that in this century, the beginnings of a great theory of human behavior were begun by B.F.Skinner, Ph.D. Skinner has always made it a point to only discuss and test the observable — he is the first scientist of human behavior. (He is of course widely denounced, as was Galileo, by those who don't, and don't want to, understand his work.) A simple example of the psychoanalyst's concepts and of Skinner's behavioral understanding[69] for the phenomenon of gambling will demonstrate what we are saying here. The analyst says it goes back to poor toilet training during infancy — anal retention or some such nonsense. Skinner would look at the gambler's "schedule of reinforcement." A variable schedule of reinforcement can cause "addiction" in laboratory mice and in humans. If the mouse pushes a button once and is (food) rewarded subsequently, he may push the button say five times without the reward. If then rewarded, he may push the button 25 times before quitting—unless rewarded. Likewise, a human can get hooked by winning infrequently by a similar variable schedule of reinforcement. And the treatment doesn't need to take years. You just use the methods of behaviorism to extinguish one behavior and adopt a new one. You don't have to recall your toilet training for years.

We believe that many gambler's have hypoglycemia and allergies. Look for the coffee, sugar and cigarettes. As Skinner didn't measure such variables, he never talked about them.

But some, even in the East, have concepts similar to Skinner's. The Indian sage, Khrishnamurti always examined things with an analogous logic.[70] If someone came to him and complained that they wished to go *beyond* being an envious person as their enlightened friends had, he would merely show them that their desire was still another example of envy itself! Skinner would have talked about a conditioned response; but they are saying the same thing basically. Khrishnamurti even wrote a book called *FEAR OF THE KNOWN*. While everyone talks about fear of the unknown, he knew better. But Skinner, in different language, would say you could only have fear as a conditioned response; thus fear of the unknown couldn't exist as a "fear" in agreement with Khrishnamurti. As a physicist, who studied "psychology" at length, I can show that if a behavioral therapy works, it can be shown to be a subset of Skinner's behaviorism. This includes the theories of many different theorists that have denounced Skinner—the modern Galileo.

#5. The use of Ritalin®, and other drugs, to "quiet" hyperactive children. Western medical barbarism, again under the false guise of "science," now wants to routinely drug children! Though Dr. Feingold made the allergy-hyperactivity connection known to the public, allergy as a cause of hyperactivity in children appeared in the literature over 60 years ago. (It was then called the "tension-fatigue" syndrome.) In fact, the work was more accurate then, as any allergy was stated to potentially cause this problem. Feingold unfortunately concentrated on salicylates almost exclusively. The psychiatric orthodoxy knows well that allergy causes hyperactivity and uses this knowledge to perform phony studies which purport to support drug therapy and "prove" allergy is not involved. Doctored studies (passing for Science) have children placed on diets either without complete omission of salicylates or else the diet is high in sugar and other *known* behavior-altering foods. Here again is the concerted effort by the medical and psychiatric professions to cover up the knowledge that people can get well *by themselves*, without toxic, drug therapy — simply by ascertaining and eliminating allergens. The callous way children are used as pawns by psychiatrists for their own financial and reputational gain speaks for itself. Here *parents* and *school teachers* are encouraged to aid in the wholesale drugging of a generation. Horrible side effects to the brain are always underestimated. And the brainwashing that drugs are the *only* therapy is ingrained in the parent, school teacher and the child.

#6. "Psychosurgery." We put this in quotes as it is another misnomer. The "psyche" is not being operated on, the brain is! This primarily includes the various lobotomy operations — they sever or destroy the corpus callosum, which you recall, connects the two brain hemispheres. Here without any scientific support, the communication between the two fundamental halves of a person's being is permanently destroyed (again under the false guise of "science"). This operation has been used when ECT was ineffective, when aberrant behavior couldn't be otherwise stifled and today when drugs fail to stop epileptic seizures. We note that anti-epileptic drugs will fail if the cause of the seizures are ecological or nutritional. The sad thing is that more enlightened M.D.'s have written research books on how various nutrients, like the amino acid, taurine, are effective in stopping seizures.

#7. The entire use of drugs in psychiatry. Such use is clearly an admission that there is a biochemical anomaly in the brain. But a true science would demand not a drugging of the population, but the ascertaining of the cause of the biochemical defect. And depression, anxiety, paranoia, schizophrenia, autism, anorexia and virtually all other "mental" ills have been proven by clinical ecologists and medical nutritionists to have ecological and nutritional causation. The use of drugs is thus patently unscientific. The horrible side effects of "psychoactive" drugs are beginning to become known to the population. These include facial ticks, muscle tremblings and immune suppression as well as zombie-like behavior. That such drugs won't work is also clear from the ecology knowledge, viz. the allergic person will also become allergic to *these drugs* as he takes them everyday! (Valium® is well known to lead to excitability, not tranquility, in many, after days or weeks of use.) So, just another toxin has been added to an already overloaded system.

#8. "It must be mental." The phrase that every ecologically ill person (including physicians) has had said to him or her. Again it implies the physician saying it possesses all and ultimate medical knowledge of "physical" illness. It is usually said even if there is no emotional history to support it and even if such a history isn't checked for. It is a cover-up for ignorant and intellectually lazy physicians. These are the real quacks! Patients are thus forced to either submit to a psychiatrist's whimsical treatments or seek the answers themselves. Other variants are "it's due to stress" or "it's psychosomatic." The same objections as above apply here. "Somatopsychic" would be a more accurate term as the causal relationship is closer to the truth when stated this way. But even "somatopsychic" is a misnomer as it implies a *separation* of "psyche" from the body. But the "psyche" is really the brain which is a part of the body. This last fact again is being alluded to by psychiatrists as they use brain altering chemicals more and more.

#9. "Talk therapy" works at least as well as "psychotherapy." Studies have shown that just talking about your problems to a friend or relative corrects emotional ills at least as well as (and a lot quicker than) psychoanalysis. And if there is no friend available, experts with Ph.D.'s or M.S.W.'s can be of benefit without the possibility of being drugged or shocked or lobotomized. We shall see that if there is truly an emotional problem, muscle testing and energy balancing offers the best and quickest solutions.

The reader also needs to be aware of some cute myths available from some therapists. They are just as inaccurate and ultimately harmful to anyone in desperate need of getting physically and emotionally well.

We'll list a few *PSYCHOLOGICAL MYTHS*   now.

#1. If you aren't well after a treatment or balancing, you (at a "deep level") wish to remain sick. Translation: this "holistic" practitioner doesn't know enough to help you!

#2. Your illness or addiction exists because of a lack of self-love. If a lack of self-love exists, the actual order is reversed. For example, food addiction is a powerful *physical* force. Through a lack of knowledge of allergy, a person may be unable to stop eating foods that are harmful to him. He may *then* feel frustrated and lose self-esteem and self-love.

#3. People are sick because they "choose" to be sick. This is the height of antiquated nonsense. "Choice" is big these days. It's an easy way out again. Here's an example. It's well known that the last people to listen to you—or allow you to help them—are your family members. Now my father's three packs of cigarettes a day caused him to suffer various ills for years. I tried explaining, pleading and screaming! I've begged him for years to choose life and give up his poisons over cigarettes, illness and death. But, of course, there is no choosing going on here. It's a simple, but very powerful, physical addiction and he was *incapable of making a choice*! In his case, the coffee that started off his day began a downward, daily spiral of hypoglycemia and allergy/addiction that overrides any aspect of his being that might have theoretically wanted to "choose" life. Because it's not yet talked about on TV, he didn't recognize what a powerful, addictive drug coffee is. Choice sounds great but much of the time it is a meaningless concept as much of the history of the world and most of our own histories indicate. We don't exist independent of physical, chemical and behavioral forces.

These popular notions are really a regurgitation of the ancient "homunculus" [little man] theories. These theories (like Freud's models) say, in essence, that the "big man" does something because the "little man" inside directs it. They are worthless because a scientist would then ask, what causes the little man to direct it? So you see they are not explanations at all. Many holistic physicians and kinesiologists say that emotions cause all illness. This keeps them from having to learn of the complexities of ecological illness, etc. We've taught many lay kinesiologists the HEBS methods, but most do not attain certification because they've already been "seduced" by other kinesiology seminars with "emotional balancing is all that is ever needed". The same is true of some well known "holistic" M.D.'s. This approach is anything but holistic. It is one-dimensional, and very dangerous. Such practitioners desperately avoid knowing and using the wealth of knowledge about the ecological, nutritional and electrical factors that cause "emotional" ills. Eventually, after years of illness, their patients learn of matters discussed in this book.

All this is not to say that a true science of human behavior isn't needed. It most certainly is and we should include the chemical component which is left out by the behaviorists. As a physicist, I have found it rather sad to see that every year psychiatrists, psychologists, philosophers, clergymen, writers, and others offer treatises on anxiety. There is no doubt that in the U.S., at this time, recurrent feelings of anxiety are most often due to the PHAC syndrome. These books are likely written by coffee drinkers who don't understand themselves at all! The marked effects that faulty blood sugar levels (and adrenal involvement), Parasitosis, allergies, Candidiasis, nutritional deficiencies, etc. have on the brain and thus behavior have been scientifically proven. These are the causes of faulty brain chemistry that the psychiatric profession would attempt to correct with more allergic, toxic compounds — drugs. That drugs are used extensively during the last two decades indirectly signals that psychiatrists finally recognize that mental models are incapable of describing "mental" diseases. At last, the mind/brain is being viewed as a physical organ. Soon, the evidence will force a realization that the brain is the body's most sensitive organ to ecological and nutritional imbalance.

Both the people and the psychological community must be educated to *first* look for ecological, nutritional and energy factors when "emotional" symptoms occur. And again since we have shown that drugs, shock therapy and "psychosurgery" are unscientific and barbaric, there is no need to see a psychiatrist unless he is also a clinical ecologist. But if a professional is sought in the psychological community, make sure that the nonsense of Freud and other later "analysts" is avoided too. Be wary also of many misconceptions found in "holistic health." There is a tendency here for many to proclaim that "emotions cause all illness." Cancer and heart disease are included here. We have demonstrated that this is not so. Before this century, cancer and CVD were virtually unknown despite the fact that emotional stressors were far greater. At the present time many Americans aren't troubled by war, famine, high infant (and bearing mother) mortality. Thus there is much less serious emotional stress today than earlier when cancer and degenerative diseases didn't exist. Also, you can look at many very (emotionally) balanced yogis with bloated bellies. There, sugar is often regarded as a "pure white substance." Apparently, emotional balance does not prevent Candida-caused bloating!

It is, of course, an important issue in disease to ascertain whether emotional stress is the cause, the result, or the concomitant of biochemical imbalance in the body. The history of Western Medicine reveals that whenever a disease's etiology was uncertain, emotions had to be the cause. Tuberculosis had its "emotional profile" 100 years ago. And today cancer patients are said to succumb if they have a certain (depressed) emotional profile. But recently, such depression was found to be caused by chemicals secreted by the tumor itself! (See Ref. 45.) When studied properly, chronic, emotional imbalance is usually found to be a result of biochemical imbalance. Indeed you may know someone who has lived through many terrible experiences yet is always cheerful. Why can someone govern a nation without succumbing to the "stress" yet another finds it "too stressful" to step outdoors? Clearly, it is the person's biochemistry and energy circuits, not the stress level that is often at fault. This is analogous to the realization that the immune system, not the germ, is usually the more important issue in who becomes ill. Nonetheless, the "mind" can make any complaint better or worse. And most of us through ignorance, make things worse. But now we'll start to reverse this effect. In fact, we shall see that MBT and energy balancing affords the most rapid way to uncover an emotional problem and to correct it!

The first energy "circuit" to check for goes by many names. It's been variously called *TIBETAN ENERGY, FIGURE "8" ENERGY, OVER-ENERGY or "PSYCHOLOGICAL REVERSAL."* We believe they are all the same (or at least related.) The Tibetans found, thousands of years ago that energy flows in figure "8" patterns around the body. More recently kinesiologists and psychologists have found that an imbalance here can result in over-energy or "psychological reversal." You should perhaps test and correct this even before doing the unswitching of Ch. 9. This "reversal" can exist in a general sense or for specific emotional issues.

OVERENERGY TEST

1. We can test this, in the general sense, by muscle testing immediately after the subject says, "I want to be well."
2. Then test him saying, "I want to be sick."
3. The first quote should test strong, the second one, weak.

Here we are using MBT as a true feedback mechanism. If balanced, a strong response to a statement means "yes" or "true" and a weak response means "no" or "it's a lie." This is analogous to a lie detector gauging a subject's veracity via skin cell electrical conductivity changes also after making statements. So if "I want to be well" tests weak and/or "I want to be sick" tests strong, there is a Figure 8 (or Tibetan or overenergy) imbalance. And it would be called a "psychological reversal" because, if uncorrected, it can manifest with a *stuck*, negative or detrimental behavior. But it is not truly "psychological" as the energy imbalance is not in the mind. And it's not the person's fault. This overenergy, we liken to someone who's had to work for 24 hours straight. When he can now finally go to sleep, he's too *overtired* to sleep!

This researcher discovered—in the mid 1980's—the underlying factor that caused the "psychological reversal" and subsequent phobias to occur. Even earlier than allergic reactions, it is the parasite/gastrointestinal permeability factor and subsequent serotonin imbalance!

We can correct this imbalance using several techniques from kinesiologists. Wayne Cook, Ph.D., was a physicist who first placed the body in Figure 8 positions to correct this imbalance. The following is the Tietsworth correction. (See Fig. 40.)

OVERENERGY CORRECTION

1. Place the left foot (ankle) over the right, then place your hands straight out, with the backs of the hands touching each other.

2. Then bring the right hand over and on top of the left.

3. Clasp fingers and then fold the hands and arms in and rest them on your chest.

4. As you breathe in, have the tongue rest against the top palate (behind the top front teeth).

5. As you breathe out, rest the tongue against the bottom palate.

6. Do this for a minute or two and then re-do the over-energy test.

7. "Being well" should now test strong and "being sick" should now test weak.

8. For about 5% of the population—the ones not yet corrected—this correction may need to be reversed; i.e., place the right ankle over the left and place the left hand over the right. The breathing is the same.

STOP READING NOW! YES, WE MEAN YOU! DO THIS SIMPLE CORRECTION NOW! DO IT, IF YOU WANT TO BE WELL.

A similar balance is to sit with the corresponding fingertips of each hand touching each other, while performing the same breathing. And this overenergy or reversal should be checked for all serious issues. E.g., if a person is worried about taking an exam or that they might have a Candida problem, do the following test.

Figure 40. Putting the body in a Figure "8".

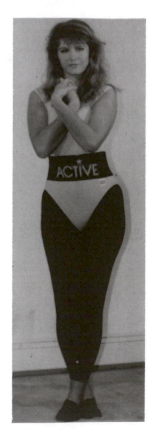

SPECIFIC ISSUE – OVERENERGY OR REVERSAL TEST

1. Have the subject think about the issue or say the issue
2. The testor simultaneously traces the central (acupuncture) meridian up.
3. Quickly, muscle test.

This tracing means the testor is running his hand quickly up from the pubic area towards the chin. (You don't have to touch the subject, just be within an inch from the skin.) This is following the body's central acupuncture meridian which relates to the brain. It is giving this meridian and hence the brain some *extra* energy. If the person is balanced for this issue, the arm will test strong. But if the person is overenergized about it, the arm will now test weak (due to the inability to handle a little extra energy.) The correction is to sit, stand or lie in the figure "8" position while (here) thinking about this issue for a minute or two. Retest with the subject saying the original stressing issue while again tracing the central meridian. The arm should now be strong. Note, the issue has not necessarily been de-stressed, just the *overenergy* about it has been fixed. Also note that the first correction fixes general overenergy while subsequent figure "8" corrections are for specific stresses or issues.

Next we can actually de-stress the issue in several ways. The first is called ESR for EMOTIONAL STRESS RELEASE. See Fig 41.

EMOTIONAL STRESS RELEASE

1. The testor can very lightly hold the "frontal eminence" points above the two eyes.

These are the points that many people and actors intrinsically hold when stressed or acting stressed. You find these points by going up from the eyebrow bone (which comes out, away from the head.) You will pass a valley which goes in towards the head. Just above are the eminences which again go out, away from the head. Hold lightly for at least 20 seconds.

> **STOP READING NOW! YES, WE MEAN YOU! DO THIS SIMPLE CORRECTION NOW! DO IT, IF YOU WANT TO BE WELL. THERE ARE NO MAGIC PILLS THAT WILL GET YOU WELL! DON'T READ THIS BOOK LIKE A HISTORY BOOK – IT'S A SELF-HELP MANUAL. YES, YOU CAN DO THE CORRECTIONEVEN WITHOUT TESTING IT. IT CAN'T HURT YOU! THE PHYSICIST'S RAPID SOLUTION WILL HAVE YOU FEELING BETTER ALMOST IMMEDIATELY AFTER YOU TAKE THESE FIRST STEPS.**

You may feel the so-called primitive capillary pulses with your fingertips. You may even feel them synchronize, though you may not. This is also called a *neurovascular correction*. And it is believed to send increased blood flow to the cerebrum and away from the lower "fight or flight" (or reptilian) regions of the brain. These points can be held for many minutes. The person may visualize a positive outcome to the stressing issue – all *without* ever needing to tell the testor just what the issue is! In "analysis" – note the scientific *sounding* name – this alone can take months or years!

Anyone can do this to themselves before, after or during a

Figure 41.

Emotional Stress
Release (ESR)
points.

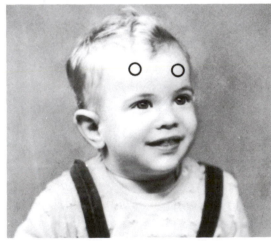

stressful situation. Kinesiological corrections usually seem to work better when someone else does the balancing—the subject can be more relaxed. The subject may indeed feel exhilarated to be de-stressed although many feel a mellow, almost sleepy-like state afterwards. Retest the arm (while the thought is again visualized) to see if the issue has actually been de-stressed.

A more recent discovery was made by psychologist Roger Cal-lahan, Ph.D. for PHOBIA CURES. The original title of his book was, *THE FIVE MINUTE PHOBIA CURE.* Callahan found, after many years of standard treatment, that no phobia cures existed for his patients. He discovered that the problem, or overenergy, was trapped, *not* in the "mind," but was in various acupuncture meridians! His book emphasized the stomach and pancreas (spleen) meridians, but in some cases, other meridians may be affected.

He first tests for "psychological reversal" and corrects it with tapping on a certain acupuncture point that we will not go into here as the Figure "8" correction works just as well. Then the *Stomach Or Pancreas Meridians Would Be Reset.* Any meridian can hold trapped over-energy. Very frequently, it is held in the pancreas (spleen) or stomach meridians. We will try to use the word "cor-rection" instead of "cure" because this author found, in 1985, that in some people, allergic reactions or *the cause of allergic reac-tions—the parasite permeability factor* continually adversely af-fects the serotonergic nerves in the gastrointestinal tract and "phobia cures" won't last.

PHOBIA CORRECTION

0. You will need to test for any specific "psychological reversal" first and correct with the figure 8 position. Reversal, if it exists, must be corrected before the meridian points are corrected.
1. You will next ascertain if the stomach or spleen (pancreas) meridians are the cause of the phobia. How do you know if the problem is in the stomach or pancreas meridian? [You could do both sets of tapping corrections without testing.] Have the subject think of the issue (testing weak) while the testor touches the point

under the eye (a stomach point) and separately the point between the ribs (Spleen 21). The one that temporarily makes the weak arm become strong is the one that will make the correction!

2. If it is the stomach, follow steps 3-5. If it's the spleen meridian, follow steps 7-8.

3. The stomach meridian begins at the notch on the bone just under the center of each eye.

4. Tap both sides simultaneously for 30 seconds or so *while the subject thinks of the emotional issue or "phobia."* (A phobia is really any chronic fear — and nearly all of us have some! If you think you don't have any, you probably have an extra one.)

5. Tap with a medium pressure, several times a second, avoiding the eye. A waltz beat — HARD, soft, soft — can be used too.

For the Pancreas (Spleen) Meridian.

7. The other set of tapping points are at the end points of the pancreas (spleen) meridian. (Discussion follows below.)

8. This meridian ends on the Spleen 21 point you already know from the blood chemistry (refer back to Figure 33) correction. Recall these points were on the sides of the body near where the bent elbow crease intersected the side of the ribs. Tap these out too.

  More recently, Callahan found that one usually only needs to tap one side, not both the left and right sides simultaneously. But you can't go wrong if you do tap both sides simultaneously.

  We can devise an additional method to make sure the correction gets into both brain hemispheres and is integrated.

9. After the phobia tapping, you can also do some cross-crawls (brain integration — hands to the knees) while thinking of the phobia and also humming and then while counting.

10. Finally retest the arm while the subject thinks of the issue or phobia. It should now be strong, if overenergy was tested and corrected first.

For some, the overenergy is trapped in the pancreas (again, misnamed spleen) meridian. Getting "the shakes" over issues or over- or under-eating when stressed, are keys that energy is trapped in this meridian. "Butterflies in the stomach" are a hint at the stomach meridian's involvement when stressed.

Callahan has been on many national, American TV shows curing life-long phobias to snakes, rats, heights, driving, hypodermic needles, ladders, etc. in seconds or minutes. This correction can be more powerful than the older ESR correction. All this points out that if the problem is truly emotional, *kinesiologists*, have uncovered the best and quickest way to ascertain and correct the cause! And the environmentally ill (and everyone else) have, or will have, many emotional stresses. Now agoraphobia (a constant nervous anxiety) is likely to be hypoglycemia and these meridian corrections won't work here. Just go to an agoraphobic self-help meeting and watch virtually 100% of them smoke and drink coffee? And they wonder why they have the shakes. Indeed, biochemical imbalance causes many seemingly "emotional" disorders.

The way the mind works can be deceptive (and incorrectly interpreted by most "professionals"). *The mind works to almost immediately attach a thought to vague feelings of anxiety that may be chemically induced!* (Some would even say it is the left brain hemisphere attaching a verbal notion to the feelings of the right hemisphere.)

Incorrectly interpreting actual biochemical imbalance for "deep emotional feelings" may be very common in the psychologically (and ecologically) ignorant West!

One example would be a son not getting along properly with his mother. A psychiatrist might make a case for "Oedipus complex." However, if the son suffered from some aspect of the PHAC Syndrome, he wouldn't get along with *anyone* who he's around much of the time. This simply (usually) turns out to be the mother. And all too often the stress of one's early years may be given the blame for some problem. This is easy to do if the upbringing was traumatic. But the individual may well be suffering from genetical-ly-predetermined, emotional disorders because of chemical and energy imbalance. Indeed, his parents may have brought him up poorly, precisely because of *their* energy and ecology imbalance!

These emotional corrections may prove handy after correcting ecological and nutritional factors as conditioned negative responses to eating, drinking or breathing things may have occurred. Indeed some "allergies" in a universal reactor may be phobias or some of the stress may be emotional as well as ecological. But, as always, we believe the original cause is truly ecological. As the "mind" *can* make things better or worse, we now have several, remarkable options of the former kind! And those in the psychological profession who have availed themselves of these methods have found them to indeed be the quickest available. We do indeed need more, not less, of such professionals in our society. But instead of using unscientific mental models, ecological and energy factors should be considered first. The professional may then need to supply support for such things as diet change, as addiction correction is a great stress. Indeed, few of us don't cheat on our diets occasionally. This author believes there is an analogous Peter Principle involved here. This principle relates to the business world, where one is promoted as a reward until one reaches a level that is too difficult for the individual. He then becomes stuck at a level he is incompetent at! Likewise many cheat at their diets, not killing themselves, but just to the point where they are never totally well. The methods of this chapter can be used to help one towards true, optimum health! Also, with these MBT and energy balancing methods the E.I can feel *well* as their ecological imbalance is dealt with.

Towards this end, this author created the first healing/relaxation tape for allergies and Candidiasis. The psychologists tell us that it takes about 30 days to change a habit. This may be due to the moon's effects on us as a woman's monthly cycle apparently is. During this time we need all the help we can get. (The one food you just can't give up is probably your worst allergy!) This tape offers support for diet and lifestyle changes and for doing the corrections from this book. It can help you to end the cycle of viewing food as a reward and reinforce you to find other things (friends, entertainment, etc.) to reward yourself with. Many people inadvertently, use foods that get them high as a subconscious reward system. The tape is available from HEBS—see the order form at the end of the book.

We can't stress enough that severe anxiety states—progressing all the way to full-blown paranoia and schizophrenia—were linked by this author to the effects of toxins from Protozoan parasites. In particular, we believe such great anxiety states are usually indicative of high intestinal levels of *Entamoeba hystolitica*. Maybe some day, those in the psychological fields will ask their client or patient with "high anxiety" if they have diarrhea or constipation or foul-smelling stools. Or if they have severe reactions (or seemingly paradoxically) severe addictions to caffeine or nicotine or sugar or wheat or dairy. These are the foods or substances that cause or aggravate these illnesses, secondarily, we have found, to the amoebiasis.

For now, you should learn never to be depressed if you have depression; never be anxious over having feelings of anxiety. This worsens things a thousand-fold. If you find, say an allergy connection for your depression or anxiety, you will undoubtedly feel much less depressed or anxious knowing the reaction will end soon of its own accord and you can prevent it from occurring again. This is vastly superior to (and more accurate than) blaming people around you or searching your past for the rest of your life.

In fact, you may have much to rejoice about. Many have noted that those with allergies appear to have a much reduced probability of getting cancer. Many people with bad allergies also appear to have fewer cavities than the general population. Allergic males even seem to hold onto their hair longer than their non-allergic counterparts.

Then there is the knowledge forced upon you that much of what is available in today's society is very unhealthy. You have probably already learned not to trust the media, the medical establishment, the FDA and other "protective" government agencies regarding your diet and your health. This alone is likely to keep you alive significantly longer than those who don't get sick immediately from their food, medications, etc. So rejoice!

16

HELPFUL HINTS: HEBS' STATE OF THE ART

In this chapter we will reveal several discoveries made by the author that can play a large role in attaining wellness for the E.I. Many of these factors have only been revealed in the HEBS Seminars or the newsletter, *THE HEB SCIENTIST*, until now.

WEATHER SENSITIVITY

The author has observed that many with E.I. have remarkable weather sensitivity. Specifically, their reactions to foods may coincide with these sensitivities.[72] *When asked to check, many clients found that when the weather was "good" they could cheat and hardly react to some of their worst foods and that when the weather was "bad," they seemed to react to even safe foods.* Thus weather conditions may lead to increased permeability to allergens or otherwise affect the E.I. The "bad" weather seems to be a *falling barometric pressure* often coinciding with a high or rising humidity. This occurs as a storm front passes by and may sometimes be up to as much as 24 hours before any clouds or rain are noticeable. The sufferer can chart his reactions along with weather conditions by calling the weather bureau, listening to radio reports or monitoring a home weather station, if accurate enough. You can easily make a diary of good and bad days, correlated with calls to the weather bureau. **START DOING THIS TODAY, DON'T JUST READ ABOUT IT!** A very high percentage of the E.I. (and others — who may not have or may not know they have Environmental Illness), we predict will have this marked sensitivity.

What may be responsible for this weather sensitivity? There are several possibilities. One possibility is the activation of overgrowths of parasites, such as giardia, amoebas, Candida albicans, etc. Some like giardia are known to be weather-activated. Giardia is said to reproduce during the full moon, for example. (High humidity, on its own will increase the amount of mold in the air and possibly cause symptoms.) Arthritics, long known to be good weather front "detectors," have an illness which some have linked to amoebas! HEBS graduates have speculated that Candida (or other mold) spores are often responsible. Some report success with HEBS balancing for mold spores. Some have lost their weather sensitivity! Ascertain and correct overgrowths if they are the cause of weather sensitivity.

Another possibility is that the dropping barometric pressure (and high humidity?) can lead to cerebral edema or symptoms analogous to brain allergies. We speculate that avoiding food allergens and strictly adhering to a low sodium diet would help cut down on such swelling. Perhaps the foods most causative of this slight cerebral edema and subsequent weather sensitivty and depression are the gluten-containing grains and sugar. Wheat may be the worst grain here. But we have counseled some people and they lost their weather sensitivity and depression only after eliminating *all* grains and sugars. Try it and let us know.

Still another possibility is sensitivity to positive ions. Positive ions can be created as air molecules rub against sand or mountainous areas. The body needs a ratio of positive to negative ions of 3 to 2. Excess positive ions, such as at the head of a moving storm front have been shown to cause irritability, insomnia, fatigue, depression and other ills. Water molecules rubbing against each other can create negative ions. Do you feel better at a waterfall or in the shower? Kinesiology can detect an ion imbalance and appropriate counter-measures can then be taken.

The MBT for negative ions—Fig. 42—is as follows.

MBT FOR NEGATIVE IONS

1. Using a SIM, have the subject's mouth closed and block off (with the subject's fingers) the *non-breathing nostrils* during the

test.

2. Subject breathes in through the right nostril (left is blocked) and out the left (right blocked).

3. Quickly test—if weak, negative ions may be needed.

   You can see if a negative ion generator or staying near the shower for a minute will correct this weakness. Then you'll know that you may have frequent need of negative ions. The first step to overcoming this problem is to do the above testing. Next the HEBS balancing and diet restrictions noted may help. If not, consideration should be given to moving to a place (like the American Southwest) where few storm fronts pass by.[73] After all, life is short, and what could be better than being able to eat anything without reacting?

   Also note that man was supposedly "spawned" in desert areas of Africa and more recently came to live in regions near bodies of water for reasons of industrial transportation and economics. But with the new age of computerization and leisure industries, you should be able to break the centuries-old "mold." Make sure to spend much time visiting an area before moving though. Your first step would be to check a good weather almanac[74] for the factors that affect you. Don't forget that temperature extremes will also

Figure 42.

Muscle test for deficiency of negative ions.

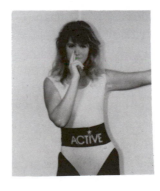

bother many. But there is no way to know how you will feel in a region until you visit it. You may be surprised at which factors affect (and don't affect) you. A final word on desert living now that I have been in Arizona for two years. It is great that there are few storm fronts passing through except during the rainy, monsoon summer which isn't too bad. However, the desert does produce excess positive ions, necessitating the use of negative ion generators! Once again, see the back of the book if you need assistance in obtaining these helpful units.

CHRONOBIOLOGICAL EFFECTS

The author has also discovered that chronobiological effects play a large role in the Ecologically Ill. Such effects refer to variations during the day (or month) of biological factors. During the course of a day, there are large variations in hormonal output, organ effectiveness and even acupuncture meridian energy. Kinesiologists have found that jet lag is related to insufficient time for energizing the meridians. Many biologists are now studying this frontier of knowledge. For example, drug studies reveal that the time of day when an amount of a drug is taken can be a crucial factor. At one time of day, a small amount of a drug may overload the body's detoxifying systems and can be dangerous. If taken eight hours later, it might have little effect as it would be readily detoxified! Heart surgery survival-rate studies also reveal a strong 24 hour or circadian variation. Many surgeons apparently prefer early A.M. operations (freeing up their afternoons). But survival rates are highest for afternoon operations! This may be due to the heart meridian's optimum time being around noon.

Biorhythm studies also reveal three monthly cycles for intellectual, emotional and physical functions in humans.[75] (This has been scientifically verified.) A date when these three cycles happen to peak is definitely an optimum time for an individual. Likewise, accidents are more likely when these three happen to be at a low point simultaneously as occurs about once a month. There are also daily variations in these three functions.

How does this concern us? The author has discovered that whether a food will affect an allergic individual has a strong variation throughout the day! When I was ill, I realized that if I didn't eat until late in the day, the worst foods had significantly less negative effect on me. But if eaten in the morning, I would get severe reactions. We can discount (as the sole factor) the saving up of digestive enzymes hypothesis because if I waited another 12 hours — till the next day's breakfast — I would get very sick again. A circadian cause is thus the likely answer for this effect. One possible cause (or correlation) of this variation is faulty adrenal hormone variations. Adrenal cortisol levels should be highest in the morning — you *should* fly out of bed — and lowest at night. I had mine tested and they were off by 12 hours. Indeed the E.I. often can't get out of bed in the morning and perk up (somewhat) at night. The alteration of sleep cycle, misnomered as insomnia, may start in the pineal or hypothalamus glands. My sleep cycle was most affected by tree and grass pollens in the spring and summer. Candida toxins, and possible diurnal variations of them, may also be a factor. (I wouldn't get sleepy until 5 A.M. When "perfectly" balanced, a delicious feeling of sleepiness descends over me at 9 P.M.) Certain foods, toxins (caffeine and nicotine) and excess salt can also initiate (or aggravate) a faulty sleep cycle.

We are probably the first to describe another chronobiological effect. We have observed that when some people go off their diet, they will begin to crave the "bad" food on succeeding days at the same time of day as the first day of cheating!

Be very wary of books that tell everyone to eat fruits in the morning. If you can eat fruits at all, nighttime may be the most natural time to eat simple carbohydrates as increased levels of the hormone, serotonin, is needed to help you get to sleep. And serotonin increase depends on ingesting carbohydrates.

So first ascertain if foods affect you in a circadian fashion. (As I look back, certain foods would lead to severe bladder symptoms, but only if I ate them at certain times.) Next blood tests for adrenal and hypothalamic hormones can be taken. Then, as always, energy and ecology balancing can help. If possible, avoid foods, salt and pollens that may cause such "circadian upset." Then advanced energy balancing can help reset meridians that correlate with adrenal and even hypothalamic glandular secretions. Recently, kinesiologists have discovered cranial adjustments (see below) that supposedly alleviate pressure on the pineal. This allows the sleep cycle to reset properly, hopefully along with a normal circadian rhythm and less permeability and susceptibility to allergens.

PHYSICAL EXERCISE is crucial to being well. It's like a nutritional deficiency, if absent from your life. Many with Environmental Illness will say "I was exercising until I became weak and fatigued." Stopping exercise at this point can insure a prolonged illness! With all the state-of-the-art procedures in this book, if you don't exercise, you may not get well! Exercise can unclog your lymph system, release endorphins and adrenal hormones, can relieve depression, put you into a meditative high, normalize your breathing, even temporalilly make your gastrointestinal tract less permeable to allergens, increase your cardiovascular output, normalize blood sugar levels (diabetics can even cut their insulin requirements with exercise), help pump cerebrospinal fluid and more.

When I became "life-threateningly" ill, I didn't know (and wouldn't discover) the methods in this book for years. Though I was fainting and would sometimes take 15 minutes to walk up a flight of stairs, I countered by beginning a strenuous exercise regime which included much running. I don't know how I did it. All I know is I couldn't *not* do it! I thought it would either kill me (physicians strongly advised against it) or cure me. And I didn't care which one, as I was in too much pain to want to go on like that anymore. It turned out to neither kill or cure me. But maybe it helped me to survive.

So get a medical check-up and if you have no cardiovascular disorder, begin an exercise regime. NOTE: Exercise may be contra-indicated if you have the potassium interference problem from parasitosis that was cited in the parasite chapter. If not, start out slowly with an exercise regime; you may feel worse in the short run. Anyone who hasn't exercised would. Do something you like. Crawl until you can walk, walk until you can jog, jog until you can run, and run until you can fly! Whatever (ecologically safe) exercise you choose, start from 3-5 minutes — every other day, building up to a half hour every other day. Then your final goal should be 1-2 hours, six days a week. Find some exercise you enjoy, whether it's a competitive sport or even dancing. Try to get your friends involved or make new ones this way.

Kinesiological testing has revealed to this author that most of the environmentally ill also do not have a proper breathing reflex. When you breathe in, your "stomach" — really your diaphragm muscle — will go down and *away* from the body. When you breathe *out*, your diaphragm should go up and in. Many people, who aren't well, breathe somewhat the inverse way, causing a great and continuous loss of energy. This can be tested and corrected kinesiologically, but studying yoga or karate, or even singing, over a period of time might facilitate the longest-lasting correction. A related matter is that many ecologically ill people have a *hiatal hernia.* Here the stomach partially pushes through the diaphragm. Pain, reflux, fullness, discomfort and breathing difficulties can arise. An expert kinesiologist can both immediately test for this problem and physically correct mild hiatal hernias by pulling it down or drink a lot of water and then jump off a chair.

Breathing problems may be related to hyperventilation which this author has found is often a manifestation of the potassium interfernece problem from parasitosis again. Hyperventilation and low blood carbon dioxide levels are often misdiagnosed as "psychological" problems. It is often accompanied by a highly nervous state but is a physical/chemical imbalance *not* a mental one.

MENTAL EXERCISE is as crucial as is physical exercise. Take a half hour a day to meditate, perform self-hypnosis or some form of relaxation. Use the methods found in Chapter 15; but these more well-known methods also prevent stress from piling up and can help to de-stress the effects of starting an exercise regimen. Don't forget the two L's: *LOVE AND LAUGHTER*. Love includes self-love. Don't love yourself any less because you have Environmental Illness. It's not your fault! And you didn't know how to overcome it until now! Laughter, including laughing at yourself is also crucial. Many with Environmental Illness appear continuously miserable, they never seem to laugh. Listen to good jokes throughout the day. Norman Cousins used laughter to overcome a deadly or crippling disease. So can you. (He also took megadoses of Vitamin C.)

Another important issue is **CORRECTING YOUR STRUC-TURAL ALIGNMENT**. If the spine, hips and the cranium are not functioning and aligned properly, many complaints may arise. This is because these structural components pump *CEREBROSPINAL FLUID* into the brain. If any misalignment prevents an optimum pumping of this fluid, the brain will be deprived of nutrients. Proper functioning of the cerebrospinal pump has been shown to be linked to the endocrine and immune system. Unlike chiropractic and osteopathic physicians, many medical physicians deny that the cerebrospinal fluid has any purpose! Here we would recommend a true expert kinesiologist or chiropractor or osteopath. All chiropractors and osteopaths are trained in re-aligning the spine and this is good. But the Environmentally Ill this author has found, frequently have *CRANIAL MISALIGNMENTS* that may need to be corrected before wellness can be attained! And the vast majority of chiropractors and osteopaths don't know how to do this type of adjustment. Indeed, some of the cranial faults, we have found to exist in the Environmentally Ill, have only been discovered very recently by kinesiologists.

Let's look at cranial faults more closely. Now the skull is not one bone, but a set of plates joined together (along the jagged lines you've seen on skulls). The plates literally move together and apart as you breathe. In fact, this is called cranial respiration. A cranial *fault* occurs when these plates get "stuck." The corrections can involve heavy or light (favored by some osteopaths) physical manipulations on the skull or in the mouth. Though the adjustment can be painful (I can tell you this directly), the benefits can be significant. Cranial adjustments have recently been found to correct dyslexia,[76] insomnia, fatigue, M.S. symptoms, glaucoma and paralysis from strokes! These corrections can work so well, some chiropractors and osteopaths are afraid to let the public know about them as the medical establishment would be very unhappy about the lost revenue. Your chiropractor or osteopath reads about cranial seminars in his journals and magazines. Convince him/her to learn A.K. and cranial adjustments. Such corrections are beyond the scope of this book. Like meridian balancing, brain and heart-integration™, pitch, roll and yaw and the other corrections of this book, structure *may* not be corrected by the diet, nutritional and pharmacological methods of medical physicians.

A well known structural defect in the E.I. is a *TMJ Problem*. The temporomandibular (or jaw) joint is usually misaligned in the E.I. TMJ[77] imbalance can correlate with headaches, neck and back aches, cranial faults, scoliosis and other complaints. Be wary though if anyone should say that TMJ or spinal misalignments cause allergies. It is likely the other way around.

Remember, this author believes that E.I. and chronic fatigue may have immuno-deficiency—and subsequent parasitosis or Candidiasis—due to a lack of breast-feeding as the earliest cause. Sucking milk from a bottle, instead of one's mother's breasts, can cause a near-suffocating response that misaligns the baby's jaw.

You may have a TMJ problem, if your jaw pops or clicks when you open or close it; or if it has ever become stuck when you yawned. You may also have grinding of the teeth (bruxism) as you sleep—ask your partner. (This may be another parasite/potassium problem as this author has revealed.) One self-test is to see if your pinkies are squeezed tightly when they're put in your ears and you open and close your mouth. You can also check to see if the space between your top two front teeth is aligned with the corresponding space of the bottom two teeth.

If a problem exists, a TMJ dentist can make up dental appliances. S/he should be an acknowledged expert; an incorrect appliance can cause more problems. Lengthy orthodontic work may be needed to shift your teeth. (Childhood braces may cause a TMJ problem.) Also the appliance may have outgassing plastic compounds and/or a metal bar that that can be a significant problem to the E.I. Use your MBT here. Some TMJ dentists have the patient sleep with an appliance that continues to keep the (top and bottom) *back* teeth clenched. This keeps the jaw muscles in spasm. Better are appliances or plastic guards that *don't* go all the way around. And remember cranial faults and TMJ problems are usually found together.

Warning: Many TMJ dentists *falsely* tell new patients that *all* their aches, pains and all other symptoms are from their TMJ. The TMJ problem itself is likely due to years of muscle spasms from the parasite/HAC condition. Your time and money should go first to eradicating parasites/Candida and overcoming E.I. with our suggestions in this book. A few kinesiologists or body workers can correct TMJ in hours instead of months as the dentists do. After going through the expensive TMJ dental "thing" twice, I got mine fixed rapidly by a body worker and then a $2.00 mouthguard keeps it in place. But allergies, parasitosis, etc. can cause it to go out again.

Don't forget to clean up your total environment. This includes allergies to foods (addictions), chemicals, dust, mold and inhalants, vitamins and energies. This brings us to energy balancing devices. One of the oldest is magnetic healing. This has become a science. Physicists have found that the North pole shrinks swollen regions and the South pole expands or brings in new blood vessels in an area.[78] Magnets placed over some internal organs, like the liver or pancreas, can also help restore normal acid-alkaline balance. Muscle testing should be used; it can determine if a North or South pole has priority. Crystals and natural lighting can also balance you.

SUMMARY and CONCLUSIONS

A most important hint is to become the expert yourself! And you're doing this now. *You* know yourself and what's happening to you *best*. You can also help yourself best. Don't wait until a magic pill, doctor or even energy balance comes along. Keep testing and balancing yourself. The methods in this book are virtually free of side effects and should be used first, or along with, any potentially, precarious medical methods. You must know what is happening to yourself. You must learn how to do the balancing of this book. Get a friend, relative or loved one to master them with you. Take the HEBS seminars alone or with your special someone. Emphasize to your special person that most people, even if they don't have serious E.I., have many of these imbalances and trading balancing will benefit them too. Don't use any excuses, life is too short. If you need to re-read this book, do so. Maybe you read it straight through, if so, *GO BACK NOW AND DO THE ENERGY BALANCING!* If you're nervous about doing the corrections, then *do them with nervousness—just do it!* You can get a friend to help with the testing. *If you can't get tested or find a partner, just do the corrections NOW.* See Appendix F for a list of the easiest and most important ones to do first—some are as incredibly simple as humming while you touch each hand to the opposite knee!

It is crucial to realize that Candida is now known to be another opportunistic microorganism often secondary to parasitosis. Thus amoebiasis, giardiasis or other parasitosis occurs first 80% of the time. And the real starting point, this author has found, is from not being breast-fed at all or not long enough; *so parasitosis can and often does easily and rapidly return even if eradicated.* However parasitosis is usually never dealt with in the environmentally ill or not dealt with properly. The author's Advanced HEBS methods —for which clients from five continents fly over—allow for immediate testing to determine which parasite imbalances the client has and which remedies will be safe and effective in eradicating them. These are then provided and our advanced, priority balancing for parasites is also then employed. (The kinesiology methods in this book are the Basic HEBS methods.) But the remedies need to be taken for weeks or months and care taken not to get new parasites from water, *UNCOOKED—washing/scrubbing/soaking doesn't kill all the parasites!—* foods, pets or other sources.

There are now so many different names—as we predicted—for the same basic illness. Chronic Fatigue Syndrome (CFS), Chronic

Fatigue Immune Deficiency Syndrome (CFIDS), Fibromyalgia, Multiple Chemical Sensitivities (MCS), Electromagnetic Sensitiivity (ES), Environmental Illness (EI), Universal allergies, etc. But the "understanding" by physicians and self-help organizations has been terribly inaccurate. It is common to read these experts proclaim that "chemical sensitivities come from chemical exposure" and "electromagnetic sensitivities come from electromagnetic exposure." If these statements were true, 100% of the population would have severe chemical and electromagnetic allergies. It is overgrowths (and subsequent energy imbalance) from Amoeba, Giardia, Epstein Barr (or other) Virus, or Candida that cause the permeability and the subsequent chemical and/or electrical sensitivities and the food allergies and the chronic fatigue/chronic pain. Re-read the parasite section of this book!

So allergy shots or drops *of any kind* may be a waste of time as they only deal with the result—the sensitivities—and are often allergenic. *Deal with the earliest possible CAUSE(S),* as we do with the Advanced HEBS methods. Find out which microorganisms your body harbors and kill them and balance the body for them. Also don't waste time and money with *bogus* kinesiology systems that use acupuncture/acupressure and falsely claim to "permanently cure allergies in minutes." Sadly, much of kinesiology is cultish nonsense with fake, testor-hypnotized muscle testing! Only if you terminate the extreme *permeability* state of the body by killing the above-cited overgrowths and getting HEBS energy balancing, will you have a body free of food, chemical and other allergies.

Remember, the author—after suffering from these problems his whole life—was helped *only* by these methods. The epilogue on the next page is from one of so many clients who was helped *only* by these methods. We're here for you with seminars and private sessions. Our tapes, wall chart, and newsletters can also help you get well. Don't settle for a *little* improvement! This entire illness is understood and can be completely halted. Yes, you can become more well and more rapidly so than you dare dream! We've done it for ourselves and for thousands!

17
Epilogue:
The Physicist's Rapid
Solution Is At Your
Fingertips

We want to end this book with the feedback from an actual reader and former long-term family of "patients" of many practitioners. You can see what our epilogue-writer was able to *do* for herself and her family with the methods in this book. This could easily be you — if you just follow our rapid solution!

"Before reading [an earlier edition of] this book and seeing you for individual testing and balancing, my family and I were not well. I was frustrated, scared and ready to give up. The methods in this book are literally life-savers. By getting rid of parasites, viruses and Candida, and by continuing some diet restrictions and energy balancing that you specify, we are well and maintaining good health. The following are the truly remarkable changes we have experienced since performing the methods in this book.

I can best describe the biggest difference for me by saying I now feel alive. Before I literally felt as if I were dieing at times. I had trouble breathing — people told me I had very shallow breathing; and I was always "dead tired." I realize now that I was in a constant nervous state. After getting rid of the amoebas, I felt so different. I felt as if I had my body back, it was now mine. I realized then that I had been sharing my body with parasites. And now I can breathe; it is wonderful. I want to write here that I had other tests done for parasites, by doctors, and they all came up negative. It was only with your advanced kinesiology testing that the big underlying problem was found! I can remain calm now; and I don't feel as if I am dieing. In fact, I expect now to have a very long and healthy life, especially because I now do your heart-integration™ exercises — the HEBS Maestro.

I have practiced yoga for some years now and the differences in what I can do now, as compared to before, are so great that people in my class have commented on it. I am much more limber. I don't shake and lose my balance anymore. Before, every pose was an extreme effort, and now I enjoy working and moving deeper into the poses. I am truly able to relax now. In addition, before in yoga classes, I had trouble knowing my left from my right. I always had to stop and think "which was which?" I was pleasantly surprised when — after having the balancing sessions with you — I didn't have to stop and *think* about this. I *knew*. Not only do I feel lighter; I have lost 15 pounds effortlessly. I don't get bloated anymore. I don't have gas. I used to have gas all the time, no matter what I ate or did.

I also realize now that I was depressed a lot of the time. I do not feel like crying or screaming now as I used to. I do not have mood swings. And I do not dwell on things as I used to. I sleep better; before I had to get up several times to go to the bathroom. I can concentrate now and I remember what I read. Before I would read something, turn the page, and realize I couldn't recall at all what I had just read! I can remember people's names now. My son just started nursery school and I have had the occasion to meet a lot of children and their mothers and fathers, all at once; and I can remember most everyone's name!

After seeing you, I experienced the longest period of time without headaches that I have ever known. Before, I had days with horrible migraines and all I wanted to do was get through the day and hopefully — if I could sleep (sometimes I couldn't) — wake up without a headache the next day. (Sometimes I had headaches that went on for days.) What a pleasure to do things without a headache! And I have found the balancing corrections detailed in your book, particularly the blood chemistry correction, are truly helpful!

After 15 years I am now free of all the symptoms of Candida. And it must be because I got rid of the underlying problem: parasites. Because over the years I took Nystatin, garlic, caprylic acid, acidophilus and followed yeast-free diets, but never got well! While I had nursed my son, I was plagued with yeast infections — burning, itching and soreness. And nothing really helped; maybe I'd get a little relief for a few days and then it would come back. When my daughter was born, I began getting frequent yeast infections again while nursing. I am still nursing her, but these problems ended after I saw you. In addition, I do not have any PMS before getting my period. This is truly remarkable and must be due to finally getting rid of the Candida — subsequent only to first ridding my body of the Protozoan parasites.

The changes with my son have been dramatic! Over the past two years, I took my now 3½ year old son to medical doctors, specialists, naturopathic doctors, acupuncturists and therapists. He had diarrhea all the time and I was really worried. He became allergic to everything he ate and reacted to practically everything in the environment, as well as having several other physical and behavioral problems. Finally a naturopathic physician said he had allergies and Candida, and this is what led me to buy your book. He underwent allergy tests and took the herbal remedies, etc. that she recommended. I now know from the kinesiology testing you did that my son was actually allergic to, and reacting to, the supplements he was given! For several months, we followed the diet and supplements recommended and he still had diarrhea all the time! It was only after seeing you and eliminating the amoeba parasite he had, that the diarrhea stopped. He had the same amoeba that causes amoebic dysentary! Indeed toilet training him finally became possible and successful after your work with him. He is now well and happy; he is quite a different child.

My daughter had been walking for 6 months, but walked very stilted and uncoordinated. This I found out is an example of what kinesiologists call neurological disorganization and is described in your book. My daughter had an imbalance with her gait reflexes. Indeed both my children had lacked brain hemisphere integration. After doing the corrections in your book, she began picking up her feet and it was truly amazing and great!

I am really so thankful, Steve. First, for finding your book and second, for travelling to see you for the differences it has made in our health! After trying so many different methods of treatment over the years and practically giving up, it has been so exciting to find and follow your methods that truly work! I have heeded your call to take my health into my own hands and I feel better than I ever have. I hope others will benefit, as we have, from your discoveries."

Helen Schiller
October, 1999
Salisbury, CT

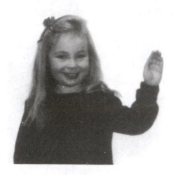 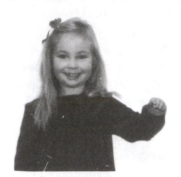

Figure 43 & Figure 44.

Casey Rhoades, on behalf of the author, saying,
"Good-Bye For Now" — *FROM THE HEART*.

APPENDIX A

RESOURCES

Here we describe references useful for achieving wellness or for attaining professional or certification status — should you wish to make a career or vocation of these methods.

Finding a practitioner or physician entails its own potential risks and benefits. As with orthodox physicians, there will be a wide spectrum in the abilities, caring qualities, knowledge and open-mindedness of holistic practitioners. We may not agree with all the methods and philosophies of these people. If you should go to any holistic practitioner, we recommend the following. Ask that s/he purchase this book (which was the referral to him or her) and learn the methods contained herein. If he or she refuses and claims to "know it all already," find someone else. Nonetheless, as HEBS is not yet a "household name," they may be of help to you. Your best bet may be a first-hand, personal referral from a knowledgeable friend. We can only hope that our concerted efforts have caused our (at present small) list of certified HEBS instructors to have as narrow (and favorable) a spectrum of the above qualities as is possible. Our International headquarters currently is

Human Ecology Balancing Science (HEBS)
P.O. Box 21091
Sedona, AZ 86341 U.S.A.
Phone: (520) 203-0689
Fax: (520) 203-0987

Please do not write to us for "doctors who treat;" while we have taught numerous physicians, few are certified. (We can only provide certified graduates' names.) You may write to us for the name of the nearest certified HEBS instructors who can perform educational, research and non-medical energy testing and balancing and can teach the BASIC HEBS classes. (Please enclose stamped, self-addressed envelope.)

This offers a more detailed view of the methods of this book. The author teaches the BASIC and ADVANCED HEBS seminars around the world. You may also contact us about sponsoring these seminars and we will send you information on the prerequisites. If you are unaware of the cause of your complaints, seeing a physician first is wise. However, we have observed that it's a good idea *not* to put all your hopes and finances in one "basket." When someone can help you, you'll feel it in one visit! We devised the Human Ecology Balancing Sciences system to offer instruction and private, non-medical sessions covering the realms of ecology, nutrition, integration exercises and kinesiology.

To obtain the name and address of the nearest certified instructor-practitioner anywhere in the world, *contact us directly* — as some unscrupulous kinesiologists have falsely claimed to be certified. It is well worth traveling large distances — if need be — to see us or one of our certified graduates!

German-speaking people can contact Certified H.E.B.S. Instructor-Practitioner,

Alexander Reichl
Ingolstadter Str. 14
92318 Neumarkt
GERMANY

There are also other German-speaking certified HEBS Instructor-Practitioners. You can contact our U.S. headquarters regarding this. Contact our headquarters regarding all countries.

Some nutritional supplement companies offer kinesiological test kits which contain samples of each of their supplements. (We recommend testing before purchasing.) We are trying to get all companies to offer this. Try to take supplements in capsule form only; with little or no excipients added. Some supplements or remedies may come in a water base which is usually fine too. The wise reader will obtain, or at least discuss obtaining with his/her practitioner, remedies cited here for eradicating parasites, Candida, viruses, etc. Recall it is the parasitosis and/or Candidiasis that is usually the first and actual cause of the allergies and the weakening of the immune system!

A truly scientific approach entails ascertaining and eliminating the cause of a problem. You can do that now with our energy and ecology balancing system. Advanced HEBS testing and balancing is obtained from private sessions or from our seminars. The Basic HEBS energy testing and balancing, of course, has been provided here for you to do for yourself!

One of the saddest things we hear so often is how people have spent thousands of dollars on ineffective treatment; or that they want someone only in their own backyard. Some people settle for virtually no improvement or for only the littlest improvement, when others have traveled from five continents to see us, or a certified HEBS graduate, and thus have had the entire problem taken care of! These latter people are *free* of chronic fatigue, chronic pain, chronic misery, chronic health problems, chronic food and chemical and electromagnetic sensitivities! *They are well as I am!*

DIAGNOSTIC TESTS

While MBT allows us to test heretofore untestable energy circuits, medical diagnostic tests are important in pinpointing concomitant biochemical abnormalities, overgrowths, immune and endocrine status,etc. Neither one is a substitute for the other; they are complementary precisely as the energy and ecology correcting schemes are. Here we will list numerous medical tests, not performed by the ordinary physician. These can be ordered by any licensed physician (M.D., N.D., D.C., D.O.) and even dentists (D.D.S., and D.M.D.). Some, like hair analysis and urine amino acid assays, can be ordered by anyone. This, of course, is fortunately the case for MBT. When you need blood work from a distant, specialized lab, just have it written up by your physician and the local lab will contact the distant lab and arrange for the special, rapid shipping needed. Don't be afraid; the local lab is glad to get the blood-drawing fees. And do buy an inexpensive medical dictionary[79] to learn the new, but very simple, medical jargon. Finally, realize that as more Americans become unwell, the "normal regions" on blood tests have expanded. If your values are at the limits, they may really be outside truly healthy ranges.

First, we know that overgrowths of opportunistic organisms must be ascertained. For Candida albicans, some labs offer a more complete (3) antibody panel test. Don't waste your time and money on skin or RAST (allergy) tests, or single antibody tests (most labs) for Candida! You can also have cultures of any mucosal surfaces (throat, nose, vagina, etc.) made to test for Candida infection. For determination of CEBV, likewise, don't waste your efforts on most labs which only perform the one antibody test which can only determine the presence of acute mononucleosis. A complete antibody panel for the Epstein-Barr Virus and other viruses including Cytomegalovirus and Herpes will test for three or four types of antibodies.

Recall for the presence of Giardia and Amoeba, the rectal smear test can be done by a clinical ecologist—call ahead to see if he/she does this—or a parasitologist. Remember, many experts believe that the usual anti-parasite drugs may do more harm than good here. But valid testing is always beneficial. The usual stool culture test, inaccurate for the Protozoans above, should indicate the presence of eggs (ova) of larger worms, which naturopathic and chiropractic physicians say are also prevalent in the E.I.

Urine and blood assays for amino acids are available along with interpretations. You may be able to have urine assays without a physician's prescription, if need be. Some labs also offers lipid peroxide assays which will measure anti-oxidant capacity and free radical damage. Also Vitamin panels (B_1, B_2, B_6, B_{12}, Folic Acid, and Vitamins A, C, E) are available.

The amino acid test will help indicate hormone/neurotransmitter status. But you can also have blood work for some of these directly. These include serotonin, prolactin, dopamine, histamine and acetylcholine if available. Also test epinephrine and norepinephrine levels. If you feel depressed, your biochemistry should show it, if tested properly. An assay of adrenal hormones may be wise. See if your diurnal (2) cortisol levels coincide with alteration of sleep cycle. Also 24-hour urine assays for 17 ketosteroids and 17 ketogenic steroids can be done.

Do get the usual SMAC-20 which includes gross tests for liver, pancreas and kidney functions. If any of the results is even border-line, get more complete kidney, liver, etc. profile tests. If there is any fat digestion (or craving) problem, you can get a complete bile acid assay. (Yes, finding a physician to order all these for me was a problem! So I basically did it myself. Now, I wouldn't have it any other way. It's not difficult to order and interpret most of these tests.) A medical dictionary (with blood test ranges and interpretations) can be a good place to start.

If you suspect faulty blood sugar levels, get a 5- or 6-hour glucose tolerance test. And don't have an orthodox physician interpret it! (See Ch 3.) Ammonia levels, according to Philpott, should also be taken, especially during the withdrawal phase.

For B_6 metabolism, 24-hour urine tests for kynurenic acid and xanthurenic acid is useful. Before any test that may relate to nutritional status, discontinue supplementation (as discussed with your physician) several days ahead of time.

Do get your immune system tested! In this day and age, even if perfectly well at the present time, a reference level can be useful later on! Tests here include T-Cells, B-Cells and the ratios of various T-cell components, e.g., T4/T8, Helper/Inducer and Supressor/Cytotoxic ratios. Other immune tests include the Immunoglobulins (IgA, IgE, IgG, IgM), C3 and C4 Complement, Transferrin and a complete blood count CBC with differential.

A hair analysis (see your nutritionist) should be accurate for toxic metal levels. For nutritional minerals, if any are at abnormal levels, you can get these tested with 24-hour urine excretion assays.

Get thyroid tests (T3, T4 and thyroxine levels) and you can also chart your underarm temperature, when you first arise, for 30 days. The latter often indicates periods of low thyroid output when blood tests fail to do so. If anti-thyroid antibody panels are available, get these tested if needed. Test any other endocrine glands that may not be functioning. Males can get a full sperm count with motility tests as urologists have recognized that systemic allergy readily affects this function! Women can get tested for anti-ovarian antibodies.

If you have much achiness, get a sedimentation rate and an arthritic panel (anti-nuclear antibody included). Here antibodies to the body's own tissues can be assayed. Medical insurance, medicaid, etc. should reimburse 80-100% for these medical tests. After having a normal screen (SMAC-20) test, I was told I was perfectly healthy. Yet when I had many of the above tests, at my insistence, severe immuno-deficiency, endocrine disorders and other problems were clearly indicated! Find the earliest cause(s) and balance your energy and ecology!

FOOD FAMILIES

Before we present our list of foods, realize that with MBT you don't need to rely on theory. You can test (and re-test) whether or not you are sensitive to other members of a family in which you have at least one sensitivity. Then too, we believe this has less importance than earlier books as Allergies and Candida can be balanced (and re-balanced as needed).

PLANTS

GRASS FAMILY
barley (and malt)
corn (and dextrose)
millet
oat
rice
rye
sugar cane (and molasses)
wheat
wild rice

CITRUS FAMILY
orange
lemon
lime
grapefruit
kumquat
tangerine

ROSE FAMILY
apple
pear
quince
rosehips
blackberry
boysenberry
loganberry
raspberry
strawberry
almond
apricot
cherry
peach
plum

GRAPE FAMILY
grape (wine and champagne)

STERCULIA FAMILY
chocolate
cola
cocoa

MADDER FAMILY
coffee

TEA FAMILY
tea

POTATO FAMILY
potato
tomato
eggplant
tobacco

peppers (bell, sweet, cayenne, chili, paprika)

LEGUME FAMILY
pea
peanut
soybean
alfalfa sprouts
beans (lima, kidney, mung, fava, navy)
carob
black-eyed pea
chickpea
lentil
licorice
fenugreek
gum acacia (processed food binder)
jicama
red clover
tamarind

GOURD FAMILY
cucumber
melons (honeydew, cantaloupe, casaba, etc.)
pumpkin (and seed)
squash (zucchini, acorn, butternut, etc.)

GOOSEFOOT FAMILY
sugar beet
beet
spinach
chard

CARROT FAMILY
carrot
celery (and seed)
parsley
parsnip
fennel

caraway
anise
dill
coriander
cumin

MINT FAMILY
basil
lavender
marjoram
oregano
peppermint
rosemary
sage
spearmint
savory
thyme

COMPOSITE FAMILY
burdock root
chamomile
chicory
dandelion
endive
escarole
artichoke
lettuce
romaine
safflower
sunflower
tansy
tarragon
ragweed

PEDALIUM FAMILY
sesame (seed, oil and tahini)

MORNING GLORY FAMILY
sweet potato

PALM FAMILY
coconut

---

date
sago (and its Vit. C)

PINEAPPLE   FAMILY
pineapple

MUSTARD   FAMILY
broccoli
Brussels sprouts
cabbage
cauliflower
Chinese cabbage
collards
horseradish
kale
kohlrabi
mustard greens (and seed)
radish
rutabaga
turnip
watercress

LILY FAMILY
garlic
onion
aloe vera
asparagus
chives
leek
shallot
yucca
sarsaparilla

BANANA   FAMILY
banana
arrowroot
plaintain

ALGAE   FAMILY
seaweed (kelp)
dulse
carageenan; agar

YAM FAMILY
yam

ORCHID FAMILY
vanilla

IRIS FAMILY
orris root (in scented products)
saffron

PEPPER FAMILY
peppercorn
black and white pepper

FLAX FAMILY
flaxseed

GINGER FAMILY
ginger
tumeric
cardamon

WALNUT FAMILY
walnut
butternut
pecan
hickory nut

BIRCH FAMILY
filbert
oil of birch (wintergreen)
SPURGE FAMILY
castor bean (and oil)
cassava
tapioca

BUCKWHEAT FAMILY
buckwheat
rhubarb

CASHEW FAMILY
cashew

pistachio
mango
poison ivy (oak, sumac)

PROTEA   FAMILY
macadamia nut

MULBERRY
mulberry
fig
breadfruit
hop

MAPLE   FAMILY
maple syrup

BEECH   FAMILY
chestnut

OLIVE   FAMILY
olive (and oil)

LAUREL   FAMILY
avocado
cinnamon
sassafras
bay leaf

MALLOW   FAMILY
okra
cottonseed oil
hibiscus
POPPY FAMILY
poppyseed

MYRTLE   FAMILY
clove
allspice
eucalyptus
guava
HEATH   FAMILY
cranberry

blueberry
huckleberry

PAPAYA   FAMILY
papaya

SAPUCAYA   FAMILY
Brazil nut
paradise nut

PASSION   FLOWER   FAMILY
passion fruit

POMEGRANATE   FAMILY
pomegranate

ANIMALS

BOVINE   FAMILY
beef (and milk and their products, veal)
goat
sheep (lamb, mutton)

PHEASANT   FAMILY
chicken (eggs)
pheasant
quail

TURKEY   FAMILY
turkey (eggs)

DUCK   FAMILY
duck (eggs)
goose

SWINE   FAMILY
pork (hog and products)

DEER   FAMILY
deer
elk

caribou
moose

HARE   FAMILY
rabbit

CRUSTACEAN   FAMILY
crab
crayfish
lobster
shrimp
prawn

MOLLUSKS   FAMILY
balone
snail
squid
clam
mussel
oyster
scallop

FLOUNDER   FAMILY
flounder
halibut
sole
turbot

MACKEREL   FAMILY
mackerel
albacore
tuna

CROAKER   FAMILY
sea trout
weakfish
silver perch
croaker

CODFISH   FAMILY
cod (scrod)
haddock

pollack
hake

HERRING   FAMILY
sardine
sea herring

SALMON   FAMILY
salmon
trout

BASS   FAMILY
bass
yellow perch

SWORDFISH   FAMILY
swordfish

WHITEFISH   FAMILY
whitefish

STURGEON   FAMILY
caviar

HERRING   FAMILY
shad (roe)

MINNOW   FAMILY
carp
chub

PIKE   FAMILY
pike
pickerel

SMELT   FAMILY
smelt

ANCHOVY   FAMILY
anchovy
OCEAN   CATFISH   FAMILY
ocean catfish

APPENDIX D

BIBLIOGRAPHY

1. Rowe, Albert H. and Albert Jr. *FOOD ALLERGY, ITS MANIFESTATIONS AND CONTROL AND THE ELIMINATION DIETS: A COMPENDIUM*. C.C. THOMAS, 1972.

2. Mackarness, Richard. *EATING DANGEROUSLY: THE HAZARDS OF HIDDEN ALLERGY*. New York: Harcourt, Brace, Jovanovich, 1976.

3. Dry, J. and Pradalier, A. "Histamine Antagonists". *ANTIHORMONES,* Agarwal, ED. Elsevier: North Holland Biomedical Press, 1979.

4. *PHYSICIAN'S DESK REFERENCE*, 42nd Ed. Medical Economics, 1988.

5. Philpott, William and Kalita, Dwight. *BRAIN ALLERGIES: THE PSYCHONUTRIENT CONNECTION*. New Canaan: Keats, 1980

6. Philpott, William and Kalita, Dwight. *VICTORY OVER DIABETES: A BIO-ECOLOGIC TRIUMPH*. New Canaan: Keats, 1983.

7. Freed, D. "Allergens as Poisons: Airborne and Food-Borne Toxins". *CLINICAL ECOLOGY*. 1986; 4:1 21-25.

8. Randolph, Theron and Moss, Ralph. *AN ALTERNATIVE APPROACH TO ALLERGIES*. New York: Bantam Books, 1982.

9. Selye, Hans. *THE STRESS OF LIFE, 2nd Ed.* New York: McGraw Hill, 1976.

10. Philpott, William et al.: "I. The Role of Addiction in the Mental Disease Process, II. On the Chemistry of Addiction"; *THE JOURNAL OF APPLIED NUTRITION*, 1980, 32:20-36.

11. Mendelsohn, Robert. *THE PEOPLE'S DOCTOR*. 3:10.

12. Golos, Natalie et al. *COPING WITH YOUR ALLERGIES*. New York: Simon And Schuster, 1979.

13. Zamm, Alfred and Gannon, Robert. *WHY YOUR HOUSE MAY ENDANGER YOUR HEALTH*. New York: Simon & Schuster, 1980.

14. "Shower Pollution". *NEWSDAY*. Sept. 28, 1986.

15. Ott, John. LIGHT, *RADIATION AND YOU: HOW TO STAY HEALTHY*. Devin, 1985.

16. Soyka, Fred and Edmonds, Alan. *THE ION EFFECT*. New York: Bantam Books, 1977.

17. Seyal, Rashid, et al. "Systolic Blood Pressure, Heart Rate and Premature Ventricular Contractions in a Population Sample: Relationship to Cotton and Synthetic Clothing". *CLINICAL ECOLOGY*. 1986; 4:2 69-74.

18. Truss, C. Orian, *THE MISSING DIAGNOSIS*. Birmingham: Truss, 1982.

19. *THE YEAST HUMAN INTERACTION 1985*. Tapes available from Creative Audio, Highland IN.

20. Russel-Manning, Betsy. *CANDIDA: SILVER (MERCURY) FILLINGS AND THE IMMUNE SYSTEM*. San Francisco: Betsy Russel Greensward Press. 1985.

21. Truss, C. Orian. "Metabolic Abnormalities in Patients With Chronic Candidiasis." *JOURNAL OF ORTHOMOLECULAR PSYCHIATRY*; 1984, 13:66-93.

22. Espy, Rene and Espy, Burt. "Candida Albicans—The Misdiagnosed Friend". Rene Espy, D.C., 1425 N.Sierra Bonita Ave., L.A., CA 90046.

23. Papaioannou, Rhoda and Pfeiffer, Carl. "Sulfite Sensitivity—Unrecognized Threat: Is Molybdenum The cause?" *JOURNAL OF ORTHOMOLECULAR PSYCHIATRY*; 1984, 13:105-110.

24. Livingston-Wheeler, Virginia and Addeo, Edmund. *THE CONQUEST OF CANCER: VACCINES AND DIET*. New York: Franklin Watts, 1984.

25. *THE HUMAN ECOLOGY BALANCING SCIENTIST* Vol. I, #2

26. Thie, John F. *TOUCH FOR HEALTH, 2nd Ed.* Marina Del Rey: De Vorss & Co., 1979.

27. Peshek, Robert. *BALANCING BODY CHEMISTRY WITH NUTRITION*. Riverside: Color Coded Systems, 1977.

28. Rochlitz, Steven. "Body Point Muscle Testing for Amino Acids: A Biochemical Link." *INTERNATIONAL JOURNAL OF TOUCH FOR HEALTH;* 1984:21-32.

29. Thom, Rene. *STRUCTURAL STABILITY AND MORPHOGENESIS*. Reading: W.A. BENJAMIN, Inc., 1976.

30. *THE HUMAN ECOLOGY BALANCING SCIENTIST*. Vol II, #2.

31. Rochlitz, Steven. "Recent Innovations in Allergy Testing." *INTERNATIONAL JOURNAL OF TOUCH FOR HEALTH*; 1984:126-140.

32. Scopp, Alfred. "An Experimental Evaluation of Kinesiology in Allergy and Deficiency Disease Diagnosis". *JOURNAL OF ORTHOMOLECULAR PSYCHIATRY*. 1978; 7:2.

33. Kare, Morley. "Direct Pathway to the Brain." *SCIENCE*; 1969, 163:405-406.

34. See Ref. 31.

35. Rapp, Doris and Bamberg, Dorothy. *THE IMPOSSIBLE CHILD—IN SCHOOL, AT HOME*. Practical Allergy, 1986.

36. Rochlitz, Steven. "Update on the Rochlitz Aldehyde Dyslexia Hypothesis." *INTERNATIONAL JOURNAL OF TOUCH FOR HEALTH*; 1986:27-28.

37. Rochlitz, Steven. "A New Form of Brain Hemisphere Repatterning, The Aldehyde Hypothesis, New Postulates of Healing." *INTERNATIONAL JOURNAL OF TOUCH FOR HEALTH*; 1985:63-68.

38. Baker, Sherry. "An Epidemic in Disguise". *OMNI*. 1984.

39. "La Dyslexie Serait Liee a une Asymmetrie du Cerveau". [Dyslexia May Be Linked To A Brain Asymmetry] *LE MONDE*. Oct. 24, 1984.

40. Bandler, Richard and Grinder, John. *FROGS INTO PRINCES: NEUROLINGUISTIC PROGRAMMING*. Moab: Real People Press, 1979.

41. Templer, Donald and Cappelletty, Gordon. "Primary vs. Secondary Schizophrenia: A Theoretical View". *JOURNAL OF ORTHOMOLECULAR MEDICINE*. 1986; 1:255-260.

42. Rochlitz, Steven. "Towards A Complete Theory Of Integration and Beyond—Meta-Integration." *INTERNATIONAL JOURNAL OF TOUCH FOR HEALTH*; 1987:109-113.

43. Pietsch, Paul. *SHUFFLE BRAIN: THE QUEST FOR THE HOLOGRAMIC MIND*. Boston: Houghton Mifflin, 1981.

44. Cantin, Marc and Genest, Jacques. "The Heart as an Endocrine Gland".

SCIENTIFIC AMERICAN. 254:2 76-81

45. *THE HUMAN ECOLOGY BALANCING SCIENTIST* Vol. I, #4

46. Rochlitz, Steven. "Heart and Brain Integration: A New Unified Approach." *INTERNATIONAL JOURNAL OF TOUCH FOR HEALTH;* 1986:24-26.

47. "Heart Peptide Goes to the Head". *SCIENCE NEWS.* 131:68.

48. Diamond, John. *BK BEHAVIORAL KINESIOLOGY.* New York: Harper & Row, 1979.

49. See Ref. 45

50. Walther, David. *APPLIED KINESIOLOGY: VOL I. BASIC PROCEDURES AND MUSCLE TESTING.* Pueblo: Systems DC, 1981.

51. Utt, Richard. "Pitch, Roll and Yaw and Electromagnetic Switching." International Institute of Applied Physiology Publication (Tucson, AZ)

52. Stokes, Gordon and Marks, Mary. *DR. SHELDON DEAL'S CHIROPRACTIC ASSISTANTS AND DOCTORS MANUAL.* Pasadena: Touch For Health Foundation, 1983.

53. Rochlitz, Steven. "On the Balancing of Candida Albicans and Progenitor Cryptocides: A Triumph of the Science of Applied Kinesiology". *TOWNSEND LETTER FOR DOCTORS* #37, May, 1986.

54. Brown, Barbara. *NEW MIND, NEW BODY.* New York: Harper and Row, 1974.

55. Beasley, Victor. *YOUR ELECTRO-VIBRATORY BODY, 3rd Ed.* Boulder Creek: University of the Trees Press, 1979.

56. Schaumberg, Herbert et al. "Sensory Neuropathy from Pyridoxine Abuse." *THE NEW ENGLAND JOURNAL OF MEDICINE;* 1983, 309:445-7

57. Morrison, R.T. and Boyd, R.N. *ORGANIC CHEMISTRY 4th Ed.* Boston: Allyn and Bacon, 1983.

58. Philpott, William and Katherine: "Principles of Bio-Ecologic Medicine"; *JOURNAL OF ORTHOMOLECULAR PSYCHIATRY,* 1982 11:208-215.

59. Chaitow, Leon. *AMINO ACIDS IN THERAPY.* New York: Thorsons Publishers, 1985.

60. Goodheart, Robert and Shils, Maurice. *MODERN NUTRITION IN HEALTH AND DISEASE: DIETOTHERAPY. 5TH ED.* Philadelphia: Lea & Febiger 1976.

61. Pangborn, Jon and Philpott, William. "Chemical Aspects of Hyperammonemia Observed During Bio-Ecologic Diagnosis and Treatment"; Institute for Bio-Ecologic Medicine. Miami, 1982.

62. Philpott, William. Colloquium before the New York Academy of Sciences. June, 1983.

63. *THE HUMAN ECOLOGY BALANCING SCIENTIST* Vol. I, #1

64. Rochlitz, Steven. "Is Kinesiology Scientific, Is Western Medicine Scientific?" *TOWNSEND LETTER FOR DOCTORS.* Feb., 1988.

65. Dresden, Max. "Reflections On Fundamentality and Complexity". INSTITUTE OF THEORETICAL PHYSICS, State University of New York at Stony Brook.

66. Prigogine, Ilya. *ORDER OUT OF CHAOS: MAN'S NEW DIALOGUE WITH NATURE.* New York: Bantam Books, 1984

67. Illich, Ivan. *MEDICAL NEMESIS: THE EXPROPRIATION OF HEALTH.* New York: Bantam Books, 1977.

68. Gross, Martin L. *THE PSYCHOLOGICAL SOCIETY.* New York: Simon and Schuster, 1978.

69. Skinner, B.F. *SCIENCE AND HUMAN BEHAVIOR*. New York: Macmillan Co., 1953.

70. Krishnamurti, J. *COMMENTARIES ON LIVING: THIRD SERIES*. Wheaton: Theosophical Publishing House, 1967.

71. Callahan, Roger. *HOW EXECUTIVES OVERCOME THE FEAR OF PUBLIC SPEAKING*. Wilmington: Enterprise Publishing, 1985

72. *THE HUMAN ECOLOGY BALANCING SCIENTIST* Vol. II, #1

73. Carlisle, Norman and Madalyn. *WHERE TO LIVE FOR YOUR HEALTH*. New York: Harcourt, Brace, Jovanovich, 1980.

74. Boyer, Richard and Savageau, David. *PLACES RATED ALMANAC*. Chicago: Rand McNally, 1981.

75. Cohen, Daniel. *BIORHYTHMS IN YOUR LIFE*. Greenwich: Fawcett Publications, 1976.

76. Ferreri, Carl and Wainwright, Richard. *BREAKTHROUGH FOR DYSLEXIA AND LEARNING DISABILITIES*. Pompano Beach: Exposition Press, 1984.

77. Gelb, Harold. *KILLING PAIN WITHOUT PRESCRIPTION*. Harper & Row, 1982.

78. Davis, Albert Roy and Walter C. *THE MAGNETIC EFFECT*. Smithtown: Exposition Press, 1980.

79. Rothenberg, Robert. *THE NEW AMERICAN MEDICAL DICTIONARY*. New York: Signet, 1975.

A. Scheim, David E. *CONTRACT ON AMERICA: THE MAFIA ASSASSINATION OF PRESIDENT KENNEDY*. New York: Zebra Books, 1988.

B. "NEWS FROM NATUROPATHS" in *THE HUMAN ECOLOGY BALANCING SCIENTIST* Vol. 2, No.2 Sept. 1988.

C. "MORE ON ASPARTAME AS BRAIN KILLER" *THE HUMAN ECOLOGY BALANCING SCIENTIST* Vol. 2, No.2 Sept. 1988.

D. *WHOLEMIND*, August 1988.

E. "NEW STUDY ON THE DANGERS OF ASPARTAME" *THE HUMAN ECOLOGY BALANCING SCIENTIST* Vol. 2, No. 4 March 1989.

F. *JOURNAL OF APPLIED NUTRITION*. Vol. 40, No. 2.

G. "VERIFICATION OF TENET OF ROCHLITZ ALDEHYDE DYSLEXIA HYPOTHESIS" *THE HUMAN ECOLOGY BALANCING SCIENTIST* Vol. 2, No. 3. Jan. 1989.

H. Karl, Peter. "Acetaldehyde Production And Transfer By The Perfused Placental Cotyledon." *SCIENCE*, Oct. 14. 1988.

See the end of Appendix F for new references for the third edition.

APPENDIX E

LIST OF ABBREVIATIONS

A.A.—Amino Acid
A.K.—Applied Kinesiology
AIDS—Acquired Immune Deficiency Disease
App.—Appendix
B.I.—Brain Integration
C.A.—Candida Albicans
C.C.—Cross Crawl
CEBV—Chronic Epstein-Barr Virus
CFS—Chronic Fatigue Syndrome
Ch.—Chapter
C.L.—Circuit Lock
CMV—Cytomegalovirus
CVD—Cardiovascular Disease
EBV—Epstein-Barr Virus
ECT—Electroconvulsive Therapy (shock treatment)
EFA—Essential Fatty Acid (Vit. F)
E.g.—For example (Latin)
E.I.—Ecological Illness (or ecologically ill)
EPA or Max EPA—Eicosapentanoic Acid, a fatty acid
ESR—Emotional Stress Release
G.I.—Gastrointestinal (stomach & intestines)
GTT—Glucose (Blood Sugar) Tolerance Test
H_2—Histamine type-2 receptor
HAC—Hypoglycemia, Allergies, Candida
HCG—Human Choriogonadotrophic (hormone)
HEBS or H.E.B.S.—Human Ecology Balancing Sciences, Inc.
H.E.&E.B.S.—*The Human Ecology & Energy Balancing Scientist*
(Newsletter)
H.I.—Heart Integration
HIV—Human Immunodeficiency (AIDS) Virus

IC—Ileocecal Valve
K27—Kidney (Acupuncture Meridian) Point 27
LCD—Liquid Crystal Display
LD-50—Lethal Dose-50
MBT—Muscle Biofeedback Testing
M.E.—Myalgic Encephalomyelitis (a viral E.I.)
M.S.—Multiple Sclerosis
P-5-P—Pyridoxal-5-Phosphate (form of Vit. B_6)
P.C.—Progenitor cryptocides
pH—acid-alkaline measure
PG or PE—Prostaglandin
PMS (or PMT)—Premenstrual Syndrome (or Tension)
PRY—Pitch, Roll, Yaw
RADH—Rochlitz Aldehyde Dyslexia Hypothesis
RDD—Rotary Diversified Diet
SAD—Seasonal Affected Disorder
Sp21—Spleen 21 Acupuncture Point
TSS—Toxic Shock Syndrome
TFH—Touch For Health (form of Kinesiology)
TMJ—Temporomandibular (Jaw) Joint
Vit.—Vitamin

APPENDIX F—
THIRD EDITION UPDATE, SUMMARY & WHAT TO DO NOW!

Here in the third edition, we will describe 1. recent discoveries of practical benefit to you, 2. what you need to do *now* to get well and 3. what you need to eat (and not eat) *now*. This—along with the two lists ("allergy/organism link" and the "causes of fatigue")—will also function as a quick summary of the book for the first time. New references appear at the end of this appendix.

Just as has been the case for universal allergies and Candidiasis, some "experts" are now claiming to cure Chronic Fatigue Syndrome (CFS or CEBV). They often take up to $50,000 from patients over a year or two of ineffective, and sometimes harmful "treatment." Take no supplements or remedies from any one—even the "biggest name" doctors—without some form of allergy testing of these supplements or remedies first! We can perhaps work with your doctor. Don't be among the thousands made *worse* by promises of quick, pill, "holistic" cures and other ineffective treatments! Most people can't overcome allergies, hypoglycemia, Candidiasis and CFS until they perform the corrections in this book!

WHAT TO EAT

TEST ALL FOODS BEFORE EATING. Be honest with yourself! Admit your allergy/addictions *now*—they're anything you eat often, especially everyday! Yes, even if these foods were *once* O.K. Craving something "bad" often means you already ate something wrong. Any food that gets you high will lay you low soon after! Self-honesty again! Eat different fish (baked or broiled—plain, hopefully from waters without heavy metals like mercury), lots of different green vegetables (organic, if possible), millet and maybe rice. Add to these foods (from Appendix C) so you won't be eating the same foods too often. Eliminate *all* dairy products, wheat, corn, beef, sugar, most fruits—*if not all*—for a while, tomatoes, all fried, processed, restaurant, and microwaved food, all foods with yeast and mold (see page 74). Some need to eliminate rye, barley, and oats.

WHAT TO DO *NOW*

You must start doing the HEBS "Energy Balancing Techniques!" You can start with the HEBS Brain Integration Exercise which is as simple as humming while touching each hand to the opposite knee! This is easy, so get started now! Then do the HEBS Maestro, next unravel your ears and rub your gait points on your feet. You'll feel better *immediately!* Then do as many of the others as you can.

Start exercising immediately—slowly and with a physician's O.K. if needed—and occupy yourself with good hobbies. You should try to find a kinesiology partner. You must become honest with yourself. *If you are not doing the corrections, food allergies aren't your worst problem.* Rather your own hang-ups, anxieties and limitations are stopping you from getting well! There may be little love present if your spouse, parent, child, relatives or friends won't start doing MBT on you. You may write to us for guidance. *First*, though, do the corrections on yourself *without testing*—they can't hurt you even if you don't need them! So there is no excuse—break your bad habits even if it "hurts!"

The most insidious symptom—not talked about by anyone until now—is the complete paralysis of initiative on the part of the chronically, ecologically ill. You must overcome this aspect of depression. Attack your depression on all fronts. Start eating foods that won't cause depression as a withdrawal symptom. Stop watching TV which has just been found to cause depression. Acquire good, new friends. Learn meditation, or relaxation methods. *Change and take charge!*

TYPE OF ALLERGY—MICRO-ORGANISM LINK
Only Chemical Allergies Implies CEBV (or Other Virus)
Only Food Allergies Implies Eat Them Too Often
Only Pollen Allergies Implies Candidiasis
Universal Allergies Implies Candidiasis

This list is both simple and remarkable in what it includes. The key factor is the word "only." If you *truly* have *only* chemical allergies and are sure you do not have any pollen or food allergies, a chronic virus may be the cause. Having *only* pollen allergies implies Candidiasis and having *only* food allergies and no chemical or pollen allergies implies that you may be eating those foods too often. Having all types of allergies implies Candidiasis (possibly accompanied by CEBV). This is not a substitute for proper testing.

Is Your Fatigue Due to Hypoglycemia, Allergies, Candidiasis or Epstein-Barr (or other) Virus?
THREE FACTORS
1. Distinguishing complaints
2. Type(s) of allergy present
3. Types of cravings or addictions

In more detail, this book can help you determine which of the four possible causors (in the paragraph title) may be causing your fatigue—the most common complaint of all. Distinguishing complaints (#1) tells you to look for non-fatigue complaints that are specific to each of the four possible title causors. For example, the CEB Virus usually causes swollen lymph nodes, while the other causors probably do not. The type of allergy (#2) means to use the allergy/micro-organism link (see above.) The third factor relates the type of foods you are addicted to, with the possible cause(s) of your fatigue. If you have *only* hypoglycemia, your cravings will include sweets (and perhaps some other) allergies. If Candidiasis is present, in addition to sweets, you will crave foods with yeast and mold. Addiction to foods in other categories implies allergies.

THIRD EDITION UPDATE

The following are recent discoveries, or verifications of some of our findings. First off, a medical study[1] has recently found Nystatin® to be ineffective for most cases of chronic or systemic Candidiasis. Hopefully people will learn not to trust some medical "experts'" books which promise quick "magic bullet" cures. For Chronic Fatigue Sufferers, our exhortation to exercise has been verified by a medical physician's findings on hundreds of CFS patients.[2] Former patients have described adverse reactions to some ecologists' treatments[3,4].

If you've been sick for a while with E.I. you might want to know that watching TV has been found to leave people more depressed in the long run[5]. Furthermore, the federal government has finally begun to admit the dangers of electromagnetic fields[6]. Those who suffer bladder frequency from taking Vitamin C—a rampant problem despite medical nutritionists' claims—will want to test and then try the new Ester-C® form (without bioflavonoids.) Women will want to know that frequent douching has been found to cause health problems[8]. If, like me, you suffered from car-sickness or other forms of poor balance, you will be fascinated to find that an Air Force study has found that motion sickness may be a type of mild form of epilepsy[9]. The Rochlitz Integration Exercises have also been "in the news" lately. Heart Integration has helped one person to survive a heart attack[10] and one child to overcome "minimal brain damage[11]."

THIRD EDITION BIBLIOGRAPHY

Note: *HE&EBS* stands for *The Human Ecology & Energy Balancing Scientist.* See the back pages for information on how to order this newsletter.

1. Dismukes, et al. "A Randomized, Double-Blind Trial of Nystatin® Therapy For the Candidiasis Hypersensitivity Syndrome." Dec. 20, 1990 *New England Journal of Medicine*.

2. "Exercise Helps, Not Hurts, Those With CFS." *HE&EBS.Vol 4 #2*

3. "Perils Of Clinical Ecologists Revealed." *HE&EBS. Vol 3 #4*

4. "Former Clinical Ecologists' Patients Report Neutralization Only Made Them Worse." *HE&EBS*. Vol 4 #1

5. "Watching TV Causes Depression." *HE&EBS.Vol 4 #3*

6. "Electromagnetic Fields Cause Harm In Humans." *HE&EBS. Vol 3 #1, 3*

7. "New Form Of Vitamin C (Ester-C®) Helps Some To Take Vitamin C Without Bladder Frequency Symptoms—[Test First]." *HE&EBS. Vol 3 #4*

8. "Douching Linked To Pelvic Inflammatory Disease." *HE&EBS. Vol 4 #1*

9. "Motion Sickness May Be A Mild Form Of Epilepsy" *HE&EBS. Vol 4 #1*

10. "HEBS Maestro Exercise Aids Heart Attack Survivor." *HE&EBS. Vol 3 #4*

11. "Brain Damage Fixed By HEBS Integration Exercises" *HE&EBS.Vol 4 #3*

Index

TO LEARN MORE

Please contact: Human Ecology Balancing Science [H.E.B.S.]
P. O. Box 21091 Sedona, AZ 86341 USA
Phone: (520) 203-0689 *(928)*
Fax: (520) 203-0987

> Please enclose a self-addressed, stamped envelope. Thanks!

website: www.wellatlast.com
email: see the website or hebs@sedona.net

The Human Ecology Balancing Sciences [HEBS] Seminars are the world's only wellness seminars covering human ecology, nutrition, muscle biofeedback testing and heart/brain/meridian integration™. Learning, vision correction and other topics are also covered. This is the ultimate way to get well and/or to get others well. The H.E.B.S. seminars also provide the best methods for optimum physical and mental functioning. They're also great for athletes and business executives who need that extra edge.

CLEAN AIR & WATER

Contact us about the water purifiers and personal, portable and room negative ion generators and ozoneators that the author himself uses. They're now available to you!

THE REFERENCE WALL CHART

Our great 2 ft. by 3 ft., 4-color, double-side laminated wall chart is again available! All the techniques from this book, and some beyond, appear on the chart. Includes the only complaint/correction diagram along with book page references and all tests and corrections. With 34 photos and drawings! $39.95 plus $5.00 shipping.

THE LIMITED, *HARD COVER* THIRD EDITION

A special, limited edition, hand-autographed, hard cover text. ISBN 0-945262-20-5. 272 pages. $50.00, free shipping. Only 9 left!

COMING SOON... *THE VIDEO*

The author has begun the process to have virtually all the kinesiological techniques in this book on videotape in 2000. *Registered readers will receive notice on price & availability.* Contact us for more information. **Available now:** Microhydrin® (see page 188) & the EZ Swing machine that balances the body's energies & "zappers" to balance out viral imbalances.

ALLERGIES & CANDIDA: With The Physicist's Rapid Solution, 4th Edition

By Prof. Steven Rochlitz

Foreword by John Wright, M.D. 272 Pages, 44 Illustrations   ISBN: 0-945262-48-5   Printed in the U.S.A.

Published by Human Ecology Balancing Science [H.E.B.S.] P.O. Box 21091 Sedona, AZ 86341
Phone: (520) 203-0689   Fax: (520) 203-0987
www.wellatlast.com (q28)
Arizonans must add sales tax on all books and tapes.
Shipping: $5.50 for guaranteed delivery in the continental U.S. 50 cents per additional book. To Canada and overseas: Surface shipping is $4.00. Air mail is $10.00. WE NOW ACCEPT CREDIT CARDS: VISA, MASTERCARD, DISCOVER, AMERICAN EXPRESS.

QUANTITY DISCOUNT (Either Book or Tape)
10-19 ⇒ 30% OFF
20-39 ⇒ 40% OFF
40-60 ⇒ 50% OFF
U.P.S. shipping: $0.50 per book—**At least 10 books**
Overseas (Surface)—$1.25 per book,
Retail stores: write for your discount schedule.

HEALING/RELAXATION TAPE FOR OVERCOMING ALLERGIES & CANDIDA (60 min.)—$9.95. With affirmations and visualizations. Side A is for allergies. Side B is for Candida. By the Author, Prof. Steven Rochlitz. Surface shipping: $3.00.

THE HUMAN ECOLOGY & ENERGY BALANCING SCIENTIST

The world's only quarterly newsletter with breakthroughs in Human Ecology, Nutrition, Kinesiology and Heart/Brain/Meridian Integration™. Back issues remain available though the newsletter recently ceased publishing after nine years. Back issues (or sample issues) are $3.00 each. Contact us for the complete list of issues.

Also By Prof. STEVEN ROCHLITZ

WHY DO MUSIC CONDUCTORS LIVE INTO THEIR 90'S?

The Simple, Revolutionary Discovery That Can Make You Live Longer, Increase Your Stamina & Stretch, And Normalize Your Blood Pressure In Minutes

Price: $12.95   140 pages, 57 Illustrations.   ISBN: 0-945262-42-6 Shipping: *USA:* $4.00 for U.P.S. or USPS (insured) in the continental USA; 50 cents per addn'l. © 1994 *To Canada & Overseas*: Surface mail (non-insured): $2.00; or Air mail: $7.00 Add $1.00 per additional book. Insurance   is additional except to USA.   Published by Human Ecology Balancing Science (H.E.B.S.) P.O. Box 21091 Sedona, AZ 86341 Phone: (520) 203-0689 Fax: (520) 203-0987

Advanced Human Ecology & Energy Balancing Sciences:Towards a Science of Healing, Vol. II
by Prof Steven Rochlitz.
This book contains our previously secret, and most effective methods of the Advanced HEBS Seminar. It continues where *Allergies and Candida* left off. With 28 photos and illustrations, 100 pages. How to test and *balance Candida*, parasite, viral and other imbalances and how to know *beforehand* which remedy, will be effective against a person's Candida, parasite or other imbalance. How to test and perform   Rochlitz' Meridian Integration™ Exercises. How to rapidly and kinesiologically test for vitamin, minerals, digestive enzymes, and amino acid deficiencies. Available in the Advanced H.E.B.S. seminar only.

BOOK_____ BOOK_____ TAPE_____ WALL CHART_____ Sales Tax (For Arizonans)_____ Shipping (Add from above)_____ **TOTAL**_____ Name_____ Address_____ _____Phone#_____	Use credit card or make check/ money order payable to **Human Ecology Balancing Science** P.O. Box 21091 Sedona, AZ 86341. Non-U.S. Orders, including Canada, see information above. Prices & shipping subject to change.
Credit Card Number:_____Exp. Date:_____ Signature_____	

ABOUT THE AUTHOR

PROF. STEVEN ROCHLITZ is perhaps the world's only Physicist/Nutritionist/Kinesiologist. He is a member of the American Institute of Physics, the American Association of Physicists in Medicine, the American Association for the Advancement of Science, the New York Academy of Science, and the International Acedemy of Nutrition and Preventive Medicine. He graduated with a B.S. in Physics, cum laude, from City College of New York. He then pursued graduate Physics at the State University of New York at Stony Brook. During his five years in graduate Physics, Rochlitz received the prestigious National Science Foundation Graduate Research Fellowship for doctoral research in astrophysics and mathematical biology. He taught both graduate and undergraduate Physics at two Universities by the age of 23.

At 25, he was afflicted with life-threatening allergies and Candidiasis. Receiving no help from the orthodox, medical community, he desperately found the cause of his illness on his own. He was left in a disabled state for years and was "allergic to the 20th Century."

Not helped by the holistic, medical profession, he studied many areas of health on his own. While taking nutrition courses at SUNY at Stony Brook Health Sciences Center, he pursued more valuable methods around the world. He became an expert in the new science of Kinesiology. In 1983, he devised a simple, kinesiological method that terminated his life-long state of "Universal Allergies" in less than an hour. Rochlitz went on to teach his methods, to both laymen and physicians, around the world. Rochlitz' discoveries have led to his inclusion in *Who's Who in Science & Engineering* and to radio and T.V. appearances around the world. He has published tapes and articles in health and medical journals; and by 1995 had written four holistic health books.

Rochlitz was the first to accurately describe how Brain Integration Exercises work. He is also the creator of Heart Integration™, Meridian Integration™, Meta-Integration™, and the Candida Balance™.